After the Ambulance Stops
A Paramedic's Story
David Sofi

Table of Contents

Draft2Digital

Published by David Sofi

After the Ambulance Stops
David Sofi

. . . .

ACKNOWLEDGEMENTS

We can thank Hollywood for making it easy to understand the meaning of "a band of brothers and sisters". But it really isn't felt, internalized, until you have been a part of one. I spent more than a decade with my brothers and sisters in the Department of Public Safety, Division of Lexington County Emergency Medical Services. They created this paramedic, they enriched me, and to them I will forever be indebted.

This book would not be possible without the many people who contributed advice and criticism to its creation. I cannot possibly name them all. Two groups have been especially helpful: The South Carolina Writers Association, Lexington Chapter, and the Critique Circle.

Several individuals contributed countless hours to help polish this work. Some of the best editorial advice I received came from Cyclewritr, Rainbow1, Tommigirl, Beth, and Michael Eschbach.

Cover Art by SeanShot, supplied by iStockPhoto.com

Title: Steven Malikowski (Cyclewritr)

Thank all of you.

P REFACE

July 4, 1776. The Continental Congress declares the thirteen American colonies are united, free, and independent from King George III and British rule. It becomes a national holiday.

July 4, 1934. Hungarian physicist Leo Szilard patents the atomic bomb chain-reaction design.

July 4, 1939. Lou Gehrig, dying of ALS, makes his farewell "luckiest man on the face of the earth" speech to tens of thousands in Yankee Stadium.

July 4, 1953. Our annual family gathering, picnic, fun and games.

July 4, 1974. Peter Benchley's great white shark attacks at Montauk Point.

Cowards die many times before their deaths. The valiant never taste of death but once.

William Shakespeare

Cowardice is the unpardonable sin in a man.

Theodore Roosevelt

Saving others is the only thing that will bring me peace for the wrong I have done. That is my truth.

Jillian Peery

1953- The Beginning

In the morning the sun shines through my eyelids and I remember it's Saturday, the Fourth of July, and we are going to have fireworks. Practically jumping out of bed, I run to my little sister's room to wake her. One last time.

On that day I was four months and eight days past my ninth birthday. Life was like a Ferris wheel, mostly up, sometimes down. It was a lot better than it seemed to a nine year old who couldn't wait for school to start in September, who then couldn't wait for school to end in June.

Saturday, 1953, and this was going to be an up day. Until it wasn't.

There were six of us kids at my aunt and uncle's house, and we were supposed to be working, cleaning the back yard and garage, but we spent more time running around, laughing and squealing than slam-dunking trash into a barrel and putting yard toys away. We babbled and talked over one another as we played tag and got ready for the July Fourth family get-together. There would be ladyfinger firecrackers, black snakes, and sparklers during the day, then the grand fireworks at the park after sundown. We ranged in age from six to thirteen.

Me, my six-year-old sister Jeannie, and four cousins were putting away yard tools and bikes and goofing off. The family was gathering at Aunt Theresa and Uncle Louie's house in Los Angeles, California. In the living room, mom and Aunt Theresa unfolded table linens. More family was on the way. Two dozen would come, and before dark we would all drive to the Independent Order of Forester's picnic in the city park. We did this every Fourth of July.

Uncle Louie walked outside and instructed Ronnie, his thirteen-year-old son, "I want you to scrub those oil stains off the garage floor so we can set up a card table there. Fill a bucket with hot water, then add gasoline from the gas can—and make sure the water is hot."

My uncle said to the rest of us, "Kids, stay away from that gas can; you're too young to mess with it."

Then Uncle Louie left for work. He owned his own plumbing supply store, so he worked most days, even holidays like the Fourth.

Ordered to stay away from the forbidden can, of course we bunched around Ronnie as he poured gasoline, with it's bluish tinge of color, into a bucket. That done, we paraded—a line of ducklings—following my cousin into the enclosed back porch of the house to get hot water.

Six of us jostled and crowded shoulder to shoulder into a room only big enough for three. A hot water tank sat on a two-foot-high cabinet in one corner. The tank's water spigot was near the bottom, above a metal door hiding the pilot light, a door just big enough to stick a long match through, not big enough for a hand. Ronnie opened the spigot and scalding water gushed into the bucket. The water swirled and a rainbow of color shimmered from the gasoline floating on top.

I knew gasoline was dangerous. I had watched newsreels of Pearl Harbor ablaze with burning fuel. I had seen cars and houses explode in movies. I liked the smell of gas at a gas station. But in this enclosed porch the fumes kept getting stronger. My head spun and vomit burned the back of my throat. Fear grew with every breath I took until breathing became as hard as sucking air through a straw. I started panting, trying for more air.

The room closed in. My hands trembled, my palms slick with sweat.

"Come on, guys, let's get out of here." I pulled at my sister's sleeve. But she tugged away and turned back, watching the pail fill with steaming water.

"Please, guys, let's go! It can explode!" Nobody moved or paid any attention to me.

I've got to get out! I spun around and stepped into the adjoining kitchen.

With my second step, my world changed forever.

A terrible whoosh filled my ears and a wave of heat seared the back of my neck. I looked back over my shoulder—a wall of flame filled the doorway where laughing children should have been.

I ran so fast wind blew past my face. My heart pounded in my ears but I couldn't outrun the screams. I streaked from the kitchen then through the living room shrieking, "FIRE! FIRE!"

As I dashed to escape through the front door my mother and aunt jumped up from the sofa then disappeared from view. I could only see what was right in front of me, as if looking through a tube.

I ran until I was three houses away, then dropped and sat on a curb, rocking, crying, staring at my aunt's house. I prayed for my family to get out before the house exploded like they did in movies.

Did my cousins get out the back door? Did they run into the hall? Did my sister? They couldn't get out through the kitchen because it was all on fire that way.

My dad was an army MP—military policeman—in WWII. He drummed into me that cowards deserved to be shot. He said protecting my little sister was my responsibility. Now, I had run like the most shameful, terrified coward in the world.

Where are the firemen? My family is going to die! Why aren't they getting out of that house?

Stanley, a year younger than my sister, stumbled as he came from the back porch, his screams so loud they reached me several houses away. He shuffled toward the front yard, his arms stiff like reaching for somebody, but there was nobody. He looked like a crying baby reaching for its mother.

Stanley was five and lived there. The screen door on the back porch had an unusual handle; it was a round, knurled, brass knob that twisted instead of a handle that moved up and down. Stanley knew how to use it; so did I. But Jeannie didn't.

The fire trucks aren't coming. What's taking them so long? Tears streamed down my cheeks.

My aunt and mother ran out from the front door carrying my little sister. They sat her and Stanley on the grass in the front yard. Both kids screaming, holding their arms outstretched.

I wanted to go to them, but I couldn't get up. My legs would not move.

"Why won't the firetrucks come? What's taking them so long? Where are the firemen? They've got to save my family!"

Sitting alone on the street, no one heard my cry.

"Please, God, get my cousins out. Why won't the firemen come?"

I could only pray and cry and rock back and forth.

My mother and aunt rubbed something wet and shiny on the children's arms and faces.

Eventually the fire engines, an ambulance, and my father's car raced up, tires screeching and stopping at my aunt's house.

My dad jumped from his car and ran to my mother and sister. He never looked my way, and my shame grew. Within minutes the ambulance left with Jeannie and Stanley, the siren screaming as they U-turned and sped past me. The siren faded to silence as the truck disappeared down the street. My memory of what happened the rest of that day must have followed the ambulance, disappearing with it.

The next day, Sunday, my parents left before breakfast to drive to the hospital, returning home after dark, after visiting hours ended. Mom and dad went every day, all day. I don't remember where I stayed or who I stayed with while they were gone.

I wasn't allowed to visit my sister in the hospital, and I didn't know why. Did my parents not want me to see her? Did hospital rules not let children visit?

When they came home Monday night, my mother said, "Jeannie wants her favorite stuffed animals."

"I'll get them!" Bursting with relief and joy, I dashed for the toys believing this would make Jeannie better. For me, those stuffed toys signaled Jeannie was going to be okay. And, if she was going to be okay, maybe my cowardice would be overlooked.

On Wednesday night, my parents walked into the house with the stuffed animals. "Jeannie wants them to stay at home," Mom said.

"No, please take them back—please!" I cried, I pleaded. A premonition of death took hold of me. *Jeannie knows she's dying. The animals will stop her from dying. She's got to have them with her.*

"Please bring them back to her."

I just knew she would die if she didn't have her animals, but I could not say this out loud.

Why did Jeannie send them back? It was as if she said, "I'm going to die."

I dreaded going to bed that night, petrified she would die because I couldn't convince my mother to take Jeannie's stuffed animals to her. Maybe if I stayed awake, I could save her.

At four the next morning, wailing from the living room tore me from sleep. I knew.

I couldn't stay awake, I fell asleep. My chest ached. I stumbled into the room, pretending I didn't know. My mother wailed, "Jeannie died."

I collapsed onto the sofa next to her, on her right. My dad, on her left, held her tightly. We rocked and wailed together.

Then, all feelings vanished. I didn't feel sadness or grief. I bawled as loud as I could because I was supposed to.

In that instant I saw us as if from the sofa's right side: me, then my mom, last my dad. My view floated across the room to the ceiling facing the sofa. It was so strange. There was no feeling. I watched the boy who was me. The sounds of crying fell silent, but the faces remained contorted in anguish, tears flowing, bodies rocking, my dad and mom hugging, me holding onto her arm. There should have been sobbing and wailing. I should have felt my head touching the ceiling. But I didn't. I felt nothing; I heard nothing.

A few days later, dozens of family and friends gathered at a funeral home. I learned my cousins had escaped into the hallway. Stanley was still in the hospital. He would be all right but would wear scars for the rest of his life.

We kids were put in a room away from adults. The kids talked quietly in murmurs and whispers with each other, once in a while glancing at me. I knew they were concerned, but I didn't feel grateful. I felt nothing but guilt and shame. I was a coward. I stood alone in this group, in a place where others couldn't follow.

My parents were doing the best they could, especially my mother, but their their own grief left me in charge of my own well-being.

My mother took me aside to explain what happened in the house. "Jeannie slipped in the scalding water. The gasoline was burning. Aunt Theresa reached into the flames to pull her out."

That was the first discussion I had with either parent about the fire. The second and last happened five years later, after I attempted suicide. My dad tried to dismiss my feelings of guilt by telling me death was a blessing for Jeannie, all the flesh and muscle having been burned from her hands, leaving only skeleton fingers. He meant well. For me, the image seared into my mind with screams of agony.

At the graveside, the only sounds were the drone of the priest and muffled sobs. In that hushed stillness, the idea came to me the only way to redeem myself was to save so many lives it might atone for my cowardice in running away and not saving Jeannie. My father started in WWII as an MP. When he shipped to France, he wanted to see action, so he transferred into the medical corps to save wounded soldiers. I made a silent oath to do that; I would become a medic and save lives.

That oath steered my choices of school, and later my careers, for seventy years. I clutched at the belief that I could wipe my record clean, that I could erase what I had done. I grabbed onto that belief so tightly I could choke it. I vowed I would beat Death—a faceless shadow I could sometimes feel, like being stared at or watched in secret. I would glance around looking for Death, but only a lingering sensation raising goosebumps would be there.

Before Jeannie died, I was self-directed, studious, ready to skip a grade in school.

I was book smart, reading when not playing baseball or football. Teachers called on me when they wanted to hear a correct answer. I didn't raise my hand unless asked to. I downplayed the smart-kid image to be polite.

Fourth grade had just finished when I didn't save Jeannie. At the end of fifth grade, my teacher called my parents for a family conference. "Mr. and Mrs. Sofi, at the beginning of this year, we talked about David skipping a grade. But his performance has not been what we were accustomed to. He lacks motivation. He's a year younger than other kids in his grade level, and I don't think he's ready to widen that gap by skipping a grade."

Three years passed, and I remained stuck and not meeting expectations. To begin my journey back to being studious and self-directed took a face-to-face meeting with Death.

1956- A Teenage Good Samaritan

In 1956, three years after Jeannie's death, I was twelve, in the seventh grade, and I looked into a man's eyes as he died.

Back then my family lived on a corner of a four-lane commercial thoroughfare, Firestone Boulevard, a busy street in Los Angeles County. Ours was the sole residence remaining, sandwiched in among commercial buildings. A three-and-half-foot high chain-link fence ringed our patch of yard, separating it from sidewalks and streets. Pairs of twisted, sharp wire barbs stood upright in V-shapes along the fence top.

One morning, I hustled from the side yard around into the front and stopped dead in my tracks. An arm stuck up in the air, and an index finger pointed straight up, like someone asking permission to use the restroom for number one. A fence barb impaled a coat sleeve, trapping the arm in the air. I crept closer and discovered the arm belonged to an old man. His body hung midway between the fence top and the ground.

He looked like a vagrant, a hobo. He was a decade into old age, with greasy unkempt hair down to his collar. A crumpled and stained fedora lay on the ground beneath his head. His coat sleeve was grimy; a rope tied around his waist held up stained pants. His deeply wrinkled face looked as if it hadn't felt a razor or bar of soap in a week. He smelled pretty bad, like an old, stained garbage can with maggots in the slimy bottom.

I had overheard my parents say hoboes were thugs who would steal your shadow if they could. I took this as a statement of fact, even though my whole experience with hoboes was them simply asking for food.

Torn between pity and fear, I inched forward until I stood next to him, the fence between us, and said, "Can I help you?"

Saliva drooled from the corner of his mouth, but his fat lips didn't move. His rheumy old eyes stared up into mine, and I imagined a whispered, "Help me." His gaze shifted into the distance, his pupils dilated, defying the sun, and life left his eyes. I touched his hand—mine warm, his colder.

I stepped through the fence gate and sidled toward him. He hung—helpless—so I grabbed his arm and strained as hard as I could to pull it up and off the chain-link barbs. With the sound of ripping-cloth, his coat sleeve tore open and his arm flopped onto his chest as his body thumped to the ground.

I looked around for somebody to help me, to tell me what to do. There was nobody. Dozens of cars drove past, but none slowed or stopped.

Minutes went by before a car pulled over to the curb five feet away. The driver walked over and he asked, "What's going on?"

"I found him hanging on my fence. He hasn't moved or said a word."

The driver put two fingers on the old man's wrist, then looked at me. "This man is dead." He got back in his car, drove away, and left me alone next to the body.

I stood there with this old man, trembling, until I could wave down a passing police car.

I did nothing to save him, the first person who died in front of me. I just stood the sentinel's watch and let him go. He was old and his death unceremonious. I was but the sole witness, there to do nothing but close the door as he slipped through where Death took him.

I felt no guilt about not saving this old man, about Death winning, because this wasn't a fair fight. The hobo was too far gone when I found him. And what did I know about lifesaving? I was only a kid.

At least I talked to him as he left his world of poverty. He didn't die alone. That his coat sleeve caught on a fence barb and held his hand up where I would see it was all the good luck that old man would have that day.

I vowed the next time I met Death, I would be better prepared.

And I was better prepared the next time, because it happened the following year, and I had earned my Boy Scout first-aid merit badge. To get this badge, we read the first-aid manual, attended a dozen discussion classes, and finally we had to pass a practical test, showing we could splint broken arms and sprained ankles, stop bleeding with direct pressure on wounds, make an arm sling, and keep an injured person warm to prevent shock. This badge was my favorite, the one I believed the most useful. After all, how many knots did I, a city boy, need to learn when all I had to tie were my shoelaces?

My bedroom was the enclosed front porch of our house. It was all windows and a glass front door. My bedroom sat a mere twenty feet back from the roadway of Firestone Boulevard. Venetian blinds closed out sights, but not traffic sounds. Sounds like the squeal of tires and the thud of a vehicle against a soft body. The first time I heard that sound was months before when my dad hit a big dog. The dog was killed.

So I knew what happened with that thud outside my bedroom.

I threw open the front door and there in the street was a crumpled bicycle stuck under a car's bumper. A boy lay screaming—his left leg bent in the shape of an L, his foot pointed toward his belt. Drivers in both directions stopped. Three or four stood in the street next to their open car doors and stared at the boy. Not a single adult moved toward him. They just gaped.

I grabbed a blanket from my bed and ran to the kid. Kneeling beside him, I first looked for bleeding. There was none and I covered him with the blanket to keep him warm to prevent shock. Knowing not to move him, I tried to comfort him by stroking his face and repeating, "You'll be okay. Help is on the way." He was a Mexican kid and never responded. Maybe he didn't understand English.

A woman from a nearby shop yelled, "We called an ambulance."

Minutes later an ambulance came with siren wailing. I said to an approaching medic, "His leg is broken."

The medic rolled his eyes. It was obvious from the kid's bent leg that it was broken. I went on, "He's not bleeding, and he's been awake the whole time."

"Good, thanks. We'll take it from here."

Dismissed by the ambulance crew, I strode back into my house with my blanket, triumphant, satisfied I learned how to beat Death. I didn't think this kid was dying, but he might have been. I reacted when grown men didn't. I knew the basic first aid steps. I was prepared.

Inspired, I studied more. I found the army training manuals my dad brought home from the war, and I poured over his FM 21-11, Basic Field Manual, First Aid For Soldiers.

This wasn't a life-or-death battle against Death, it was only a skirmish, but I knew I was on the right track, the track to atone for not saving Jeannie. But, even train conductors and engineers don't always know what lies ahead on the tracks. I certainly didn't.

1983- Riding the Rails In Style

Twenty-six years later, in 1983, I remained on track—in fact on a train track.

I had wracked up a pretty successful career in pharmaceutical marketing, and at one point struck out on my own as a consultant. A great friend who had worked for me was then the creative director of a medical ad agency in Beverly Hills, and he brought me in to help get new business.

I set myself up for one hell of a commute to work; I lived in Baltimore, Maryland, and worked with his agency in Beverly Hills, California. Two weeks in their office, then two at home. My first coast to coast flight started with a white-knuckled grip on the armrest. I had a poor history with flight, beginning way back in 1958.

One February evening my cousins and I were celebrating my fourteenth birthday. I was a high school freshman. It was 7:14 at night, the lights and television were on, and we were clearing away dinner dishes. A tremendous explosion rocked the house and the lights went out.

"What was that?" I yelled, and we dashed out through my front-porch bedroom door to the yard.

" Look at all that burning stuff spiraling to the ground!"

"Did a building explode?"

"What is that falling, a plane's wing?"

Someone shouted, "Look, there's a plane on fire, flying off to the right."

Then on the left, we stared wide-eyed, gasping, as a fireball erupted from the ground and up into the sky. We ran toward the center of town to find out what happened. A growing crowd near the sheriff's station blocked us, and all we could see was a plane's tail sticking up over the buildings.

Three hours later we crowded around a portable radio and a news flash.

"Two military planes, a Navy bomber and an Air Force transport, collided in mid-air over Norwalk. Early reports are at least forty-six souls on the transport plane were killed, and there were no survivors. That plane crashed into the Norwalk sheriff's station. It appears one woman on the ground was decapitated by a falling wing. A parachute-shrouded body from one of the planes crashed through the skylight of a bar, narrowly missing several patrons. First responders report the crippled bomber crashed about two miles north, in Santa Fe Springs."

The bomber's radio operator, one of only three survivors of this horrible crash, lived because he sat at the rear of the plane. But he almost perished when he stumbled from the tail section and plummeted and slid one-hundred fifty feet down the side of an open-pit mine. His pilot had managed to glide their burning plane toward a crash landing. But, seconds before reaching the flat ground he aimed for, they descended into a gigantic pit mine. They flew nose-first into a wall, missing by mere yards the safety beyond the rim.

That was Saturday night. The following Monday I boarded my school bus for the thirty-minute ride to classes. Every school day I walked past the sheriff's station to the bus stop, passing that wreckage. My school was in Santa Fe Springs, and the bus drove right past the second crash site. There it stood—the bomber's huge tail section sticking like a horizontal crucifix from the pit-mine's wall, mere yards below the top. Classmates crowded to gape through the left-side bus windows. The pit was so vast and deep we couldn't see the bottom.

We drove past that sepulcher twice a day for two weeks while the military organized removal of the plane, and of the crew's remains.

Nine years later, having graduated college and grad school, an occasional business trip required that I fly. I had no stomach for flying, and was a white-knuckle passenger. On my third flight I used self-hypnosis, then relaxed into my upright seat as we started our climb to cruising altitude.

Life is good, I am in the hands of God. Hail Mary, full of grace..., "

An explosion interrupted my silent prayer, "Oh F**k!" I stared at sky through a half-opened passenger door. The plane rocked violently, oxygen masks dropped. The cabin filled with screams and papers and clothing being sucked through the half-open door.

Today, the timing of my Hail Mary and my automatic expletive tickle my fancy.

On the return flight home, I sat in my preferred window seat in the exit aisle next to the emergency door. As the pilot revved up the engines to pull back from the terminal gate, the plane shuddered. Outside my window was a fuel truck with its hood smashed into an engine under our wing. Another airliner collision, this time with a truck, on the ground, and with me in the plane.

So it was that anxiety filled my first few commutes between Baltimore and Beverly Hills. But over the next ten months I picked up 100,000 frequent-flyer miles and an American Airlines Platinum card. I also picked up an addiction to the rush of take-offs. The frequent flyer upgrades to business or first-class helped fuel my longing for the next flight. I began chuckling inwardly at the white-knuckle flyers beside me.

A few months after starting my work commute, my secretary handed me a letter from an industry association. It read, *Dear Mr. Sofi, our annual conference will be held in Chicago in May. The main panel session will feature three guest speakers discussing The Role of Innovative Thinking in New Product Research and Development. We'd be honored if you would join this panel and share your story of how you brought tamoxifen to market.*

We had two months to arrange this trip. I was now addicted to flying, but time permitting I still preferred rail travel. Trains were more luxurious than planes. On a train, I could read, strike up easy conversations, fire up my Compaq computer, shower, stretch out in comfort. Traveling in a sleeper was better than flying first class, and cheaper. Trips took longer, but that was part of the appeal. I pictured me riding the Orient Express.

Departure day arrived, and with an "All Aboard" the Amtrak pulled out of Los Angeles Union Station. I had my own cabin with its fold-down bed and private toilet in the Pullman Slumbercoach.

I unpacked my suitcase, hung my suit, shirts, and ties in a small but adequate closet, and put my toiletries on a bathroom shelf. Reclining on the pull-down bed, I opened the book I had brought along, Alexander King's, *May This House Be Safe From Tigers*.

Jack Paar, host of the original Tonight Show, introduced the raconteur Alexander King to a large American audience. I think years later *The Most Interesting Man In the World* campaign by Dos Equis was modeled on Mr. King, who could keep me laughing until tears rolled. *Time* magazine described him as, "an ex-illustrator, ex-cartoonist, ex-adman, ex-editor, ex-playwright, ex-dope addict, ex-painter, ex-husband to three wives, and an ex-Viennese of sufficient age to remember mutton chopped Emperor Franz Joseph."

In the late afternoon, finished with this delightful book, I strolled to the dining car, treating myself to a relaxed dinner. Dining cars doubled as observation cars, with expansive windows starting at table level and continuing in an arch overhead like a sunroof. I sat alone at the first table upon entering the car, a bulkhead and doorway behind me. I ordered the Fred Harvey steak dinner, which included two glasses of wine and dessert, the whole meal served on china. Even first-class American Airlines flights did not match this.

We were traveling through the Mojave desert, and the setting sun's rays came in over my shoulder, setting the passing desert's red rocks ablaze. Stately thirty-foot Joshua Trees cast late afternoon shadows a hundred yards long across flat desert sand and tumbleweeds. An Amtrak brochure informed me *Mormon settlers named the Joshua Tree. Its shape reminded these settlers of a bible story about Joshua keeping his hands reaching out to guide the Israelites.* The eastern sky was banded orange and purple, and the Rockies ahead of us blazed with reflected light.

An attendant brought a glass of Cabernet to enjoy while waiting for my food. Aside from myself and two white-coated attendants, one at each end of the car, the car was empty except for three men and a woman eating at a table halfway down the diner. They wore business suits, while I sat in comfortable black chinos, a sky blue button down sport shirt, and black loafers. I thought, *they'll be getting off at a station in California or Arizona. Otherwise, they'd have changed into comfortable clothes like I did.*

The attendant brought my dinner and a second glass of wine. Almost through my meal, the woman halfway down the diner sprang from her seat, clutching her throat scissor-like with both hands—*she's choking!* A hot flash washed over me as my chest and stomach tightened. I watched for a few seconds for her companions or an attendant to help her.

The three men dining with her didn't move, maybe unaware of her plight, maybe too stunned to react. Neither steward moved to help her.

I've got to do something! The Heimlich maneuver! I had read about it in my Pre-Med courses and saw it once or twice in television movies.

I jumped up and covered the distance to her in a couple of long strides and wrapped my arms around her waist from behind. Holding both fists in the pit of her stomach, I pulled sharply.

Nothing.

I feared I would break ribs or crush organs. But she would surely die if I didn't clear her airway. I couldn't hesitate. Bracing against her body, I moved my fists inches upward to her solar plexus just beneath her sternum. I didn't pull—I jerked! I jerked so hard I thought my hands hit her spine.

A chunk of meat flew across the aisle. The woman gasped in a lung-full of air.

She didn't faint, she remained standing, leaning forward against a table opposite hers, inhaling great gulps of air. I turned and walked back to my table, and without sitting down drained the last of my wine. The adrenalin rush killed my appetite, so I strode from the dining car without a look back. During this entire encounter, not a single person spoke a word in the diner. I didn't see the four travelers again.

I fell asleep smiling. I had saved a life. I beat Death—me, alone, face-to-face against my archenemy. And I won with only the most basic of first aid training and watching television. Yes, I was on the right track.

I had no idea television would come in handy again only a few weeks later.

1983- Cashing a Check

Back in the office two weeks after returning from Chicago, I needed pocket money and drove to a Beverly Hills bank. I ate out almost daily while in California, often choosing takeout vendors to save funds, and often these didn't take plastic payments.

At noon, a lunch crowd filled the bank lobby. *Holy cow, I didn't expect this, is it payday?* But I wanted money for dinner, so I waited in line, skipping lunch if I must. Tapping my foot to a tune in my head, I looked around aimlessly.

Lines were five deep at all the teller windows. A low murmur of conversations floated in the room. An elderly couple stood in line ahead of me. The old gentleman stood all spindly, thin, even cadaverous, tottering forward when the line moved ahead. His wispy white hair looked as soft as a spider's web. He looked like a shovel handle wearing a shirt. The woman was thin as a rail.

Without warning, the old gentleman straightened to his full five-and-a-half foot height. He tilted back toward me in slow motion, falling as stiff as the shovel handle he impersonated. His head thunked like a coconut on the tile floor.

The shock hit me instantly, like falling in freezing water. I didn't breathe, couldn't think, couldn't even move. Then I snapped to and jerked into action, crouched next to him, shook his shoulder, and said, "Sir, can you hear me?"

Nothing.

Everyone standing around backed away.

With my ear an inch from his face, I listened for breath sounds. I looked sideways down his chest for any movement.

Nothing.

I put my ear on his chest, but there was no heartbeat in there.

My throat went dry, my chest tightened. My mind raced. *What should I do? I've got to do something.*

TV shows like *Emergency* and *M*A*S*H* were my only CPR training.

I put one hand over the other in the middle of his chest and pushed hard. With a sound like popping corn, ribs cracked. Ribs never cracked on television! I stole a quick glance to see if others had heard me breaking his ribs. Several in the crowd gasped and murmured. I guessed they heard.

Gathering my wits, I continued compressions, ribs no longer popping. After counting thirty pumps, I covered his mouth with mine and started mouth-to-mouth. A puff of air across my cheek reminded me: close his nose! Pinching it tight, I blew twice. His chest rose, but not as much as I expected.

I resumed chest compressions and counted out loud, "One two three four five...", all the way to thirty. *How fast am I supposed to push?* I didn't know, but subconsciously I may have matched my adrenalin-rush heartbeat.

After doing thirty compressions and two breaths three or four times, I became winded and light-headed. I called out, "Can anyone help me?" In my ears, my voice sounded angrier than I intended.

A teller stepped forward and knelt on the opposite side of him. *She's pregnant! The only person with an excuse not to help. What's wrong with people?*

She took over mouth-to-mouth and I pumped on his chest. We kept this up, alternating compressions and rescue breaths as if we had practiced together for months. Looking back today, I suspect we would have won Dancing With The Stars had we been dancing.

Medics arrived, a bank staffer having called 911. The old man hadn't flinched or groaned, and I believed he was gone. My pregnant helper and I stood aside, and the man's crying wife came over to hug us, unable to speak through her tears. The medics wheeled the old man out on their gurney with someone helping his crying wife walk to the ambulance.

The teller brought a trembling hand to her forehead. She looked into my eyes and nodded, the corners of her mouth twitched into a weak smile. I nodded in reply, not trusting I could control my voice. We became what Aussies refer to as mates. We gave each other a comrades-in-arms-hug and walked our separate ways.

Defeated, dejected because of failing to save him, I returned to work. I mumbled the story to my stunned secretary, who sat listening with her hand covering her mouth. I asked her to reschedule my afternoon appointments and left for my apartment. Exhausted, I barely had enough energy to walk out to my rental car.

At work the next morning, I sat at my desk and called the bank as soon as they opened; would they give me the pregnant teller's name? The bank staffer said she couldn't give out personal information, but she told me the bank manager had called the hospital and they reported the older gentleman had not died.

"He's alive. He made it!" I let out a whoop, high-fived my secretary and gave her a hug for taking it on herself to cover for me the prior afternoon. She happily filled my next request for a favor, to find a class teaching proper CPR. A pregnant bank teller and a caring secretary catapulted to the top of my gratitude list.

Once again, I saved a life—face-to-face. I kept my vow to beat Death, to atone for not saving my sister. Now, if only saving enough lives erased my nine-year-old cowardice. Then I would be free from this ball-and-chain of guilt. The last couple of weeks proved this could happen.

After the train and the bank, I looked toward Heaven and said, "Jeannie, I'm making up for it."

I was unbeatable.

2006- Transition to EMS

By the time 2004 rolled around, I had left the consulting world, left Beverly Hills and Baltimore, and worked as the tactical commander leading an NGO security team guarding nuclear fuel rods in South Carolina. I was cross trained and certified as an EMT to provide 24/7/365 emergency medical coverage for the nuclear plant. The cross training led two years later to my working two full-time jobs: days as a major in a security force, and nights as a Basic Level EMT, a private, in the County's Public Safety/Emergency Medical Services department.

In 2006 I left the Department of Energy gig, my only job a full-time EMT responding to 911 medical emergencies. I had to use a rear-view mirror to see my middle age. I was an old man in a young person's profession. There was nothing at all special about me, except I saved lives for a living.

I rose rapidly through the ranks and in 2008 was handed my paramedic certification, becoming a sergeant and crew chief in EMS.

I don't remember the details of my first call on the ambulance. I do remember the excitement as the alarm in our station rang. Someone needed me and I was equipped to handle their emergency. In reality, nothing prepared me for the horrific scenes I would face over the ensuing years. Everyone thinks before getting into this field that it will be an emotional rush to help and rescue people who needed us. But, after years on the street, after thousands of battles against Death, I reached the point of praying each call toned out would be a false alarm.

I don't remember most of the calls. But I do remember dozens. Following are a few calls that marked my relentless fight, calls I remember with crystal clarity. These stand out like pinnacles surrounding the valley of the shadow of death through which I marched. They are seared into my memory. Every day I felt as if I were in a tug of war with Death, digging my heels into sand while Death pulled me and my patients inexorably toward the abyss.

2009-A Soothing Bath

She was twenty-four, a hospital nurse working the night shift in the emergency room. Arriving home at eight in the morning, exhausted, she slid out of her car and looked at a baby blue sky peeking through cotton-ball clouds. A gorgeous spring day. She had stopped at her mom's house to pick up her eight-month-old son. She adored her mom, not just as a doting grandmother and ever-faithful babysitter.

She could hardly wait for a blissful hot bath followed by a soothing body lotion self-massage. She thought, *after last night's frenzied shift I need this rest and relaxation.*

The nurse settled her son on the bathroom floor in his stay-safe chair. He gazed into her eyes, cooed, then sucked on his bottle of warm milk. She started filling the tub, balancing the hot and cold to a little above tolerable. It would be just right in a few minutes when she got in. She stepped into her bedroom, traded her uniform for a blue terry cloth bathrobe over a silk nightgown. Returning to the bathroom, she leaned over the tub to light scented candles.

She struck a match—and the bathroom blew up!

My partner Tanya and I sat in our ambulance in a grocery store parking lot, engine idling. We were Unit Five today. On standby, we were covering an area for another unit which had been toned out to a previous call. Tanya leaned her head back and rested her hands on the bottom of the steering wheel, her eyes half closed. Her early summer tan turned her skin the color of light honey.

I stared through the windshield at a baby blue sky with white clouds floating like puffs of cotton in the clear air. Our windows were down, letting the cool morning air blow in, lightly scented by nearby magnolia trees.

It was the first day we worked together since I made Paramedic. She was a dependable partner, having more than a decade in the service, and I could learn a lot from her. No one else seemed to know why she refused to consider paramedic school, even though her talent was considerable. She hinted to me one day she was afraid of taking tests. We had an adage: Paramedics save lives, Basics save Paramedics. She would prove the truth of that again and again over the next ten years working with her.

She said, "Sarge, what's on your mind? I can hear your wheels spinning."

I glanced at her, mulled her question a few seconds, then answered, "You know how they train us to think horses, not zebras, when we hear hoofbeats?"

"Yeah. I heard that when I was in nursing school. When we don't know what's wrong with a patient, it's most likely something common and not an exotic killer virus, Ebola, or something. We assume hoofbeats are much more likely to mean horses, not zebras."

"Well, when I hear hoofbeats, I look for zebras. They're more dangerous. I look for the worst possible causes, the zebras, then rule them out. I keep on looking until all that's left is something common. When people go the other way, looking for the more common, the horses, they too often jump to the easy conclusion it's the first thing they thought of, and they miss the killer. That's like a detective trying to solve a crime, and focusing on the first and easiest suspect and not looking for other suspects."

"Sarge, I see your point. If it works for you, great. But, I think that approach will wear you out sooner rather than later. It's got to stress you out some." Tanya had recently crossed the date line into her thirties, but a hard upbringing gave her the wisdom of a grandmother.

She turned to face me and gave an understanding nod, "Well I'll tell you what Sarge, today we will not be in the zoo, so there won't be any stampeding zebras..."

Three radios sounded out the dispatched call, "Unit Five, County, emergency traffic." Each medic wore a portable radio hooked to their belt with a hand mic clipped to their shoulder epaulet, and the ambulance had a dash mounted radio. Tanya's, mine, and the truck's radios were all turned on; we had forgotten to turn down the sound on our portables.

Thumbing the dash radio mic I answered, "County, Unit Five responding."

"Unit Five, County, house fire with burns...". Dispatch read out the address which was three miles away. Every medic has top-of-the-list terrifying calls giving them nightmares—their most dreaded calls. Burn calls remained at the top of my list, right there with pediatric arrests. Fire killed my sister. Seeing burns now could trigger spasms of retching and flashbacks. I choked down bile rising in my throat.

"County, Unit Five en route. Place the helicopter on standby!"

We put an EMS helicopter on standby because severe burns required specialized care in a burn center. If there were no traffic tie-ups, the closest burn center was seventy miles and an hour away by ambulance. We flew critical burns whenever the medevac choppers could fly.

Getting a medevac en route involved a complex chain of events and a lot of coordination. Dispatch would call a private company based in Colorado that owned and operated the medevac helicopters. This company dispatched choppers from their central command a continent away. Before sending us a helicopter, they checked aircraft availability and local weather here in South Carolina. If there was a chopper available, and if weather permitted, they would relay launch authorization. Then it took the local flight crew fifteen to twenty minutes to rev up the bird and complete a final preflight check.

While the flight crew scrambled, our County Dispatch would prepare to send the closest fire crew to a selected landing zone, or LZ. Dispatch and EMS shift supervisors reviewed the twenty-seven predesignated LZs, and if none seemed in line between the incident scene and the burn center, then they prepared to look for an impromptu spot, perhaps a clear area on an interstate. We always tried to avoid driving away from the emergency room we needed to get to; we always tried to save seconds and minutes.

That's why we put helicopters on standby even before arriving at the scene, before we could know if we needed them—which turned out to be only one in ten times of putting them on standby. Flight crews preferred doing twenty minutes of unnecessary preflight checks to arriving twenty minutes too late for a critical patient.

Tanya drove expertly. She kept her speed appropriate, her movements efficient. She yelped our sirens and blasted the air horn to move drivers out of the way. I planned out loud while watching the traffic on my side. Talking through the plan helped control my nerves and kept Tanya and me thinking alike. As the crew chief, I was responsible to do a pre-call briefing with my partner

"Tanya, I'll grab the small trauma kit when we arrive. You stay in the truck and set up a burn kit and a saline drip set. Review the burn protocol with me."

Tanya said, "Sure. We use the chopper to fly the patient to the burn center if there are third-degree burns over five percent of BSA." BSA: body surface area.

I chimed in, "Yes, and if there are second- or third-degree burns on the face, hands, feet, genitalia, perineum, or a major joint. And our priority is to manage the patient's airway."

I was saying it out loud because when under pressure, people think better when they hear themselves say the words. It also ensured my partner and I worked in sync.

Tanya turned onto the right street. Two fire engines were parked a half-block ahead of us in front of a 1980s house. One firefighter stood next to a woman wearing a bathrobe and sitting on a concrete front porch. Other firefighters in full breathing gear strode in and out of the house, unhurried, mopping up after putting out the fire.

The woman on the front steps held her arms straight out in front of her, wailing. Her open bathrobe exposed her nightgown, and wisps of gray smoke curled from both garments. She looked to be in her middle twenties and in extreme pain. A flashback blinded me for an instant. There was my sister sitting on the grass, holding her arms straight out in front of her, screaming.

Her arms are burned! Burned arms mean this woman is likely a burn-center case, with at least elbow joints involved. I knew in my gut this woman needed to be flown out.

"Tanya, stay in the truck and get a burn sheet ready."

"Will do, Sarge."

Jumping from my seat, I rushed straight to the woman. Her face was ruby-grapefruit red, suggesting first- or second-degree burns and an injured airway! Her arms were blistering. Blisters confirmed second-degree burns; holding them straight meant lots of pain. I made a snap decision, *we need to fly her!*

I keyed my radio mic as I hurried to her, "County, Unit Five, launch the chopper, and tell us which landing zone we're using."

Dispatch would pick the closest landing zone where we would meet the helicopter. And they would send a fire crew to block off local traffic, check for any obstacles, and for wind conditions on the ground. Firefighters at the LZ also established radio connection with the incoming chopper.

The woman kept screaming, "Save my son. Please!"

She didn't see another firefighter in the front yard carrying the little boy. She didn't see her son appeared uninjured. *Is she confused, or are her eyes burned?*

In mid-stride, I called to the firefighter holding her, "We need to get her into the unit stat!" With his help, I pulled off her smoking robe. We each took one side of her body, not touching her arms, and moved her toward the ambulance parked ten yards away. She kept looking around, crying for her son, and I promised, "He's all right. A firefighter is holding and taking care of him." *She's looking around so she can see; her eyes may not be burned.*

Tanya reached down to help as the firefighter and I supported the woman up into the unit.

Tanya called to the firefighter, "Close the doors, please!"

"Tanya, we need to strip her out of this nightgown and get a sterile burn sheet on her."

The woman balked, "I'm on my period."

In unison, Tanya and I reassured her. Tanya said, "We don't care, that isn't an issue for us, but we need to get this nightgown off before it melts onto your skin."

Firefighters wouldn't hesitate to strip a colleague if their clothes were burning. But I encountered few who felt comfortable stripping a civilian, especially in a front yard.

I slit her nightgown open with trauma shears that cut the fabric as if cutting air, trying not to pull any skin. The nightgown slipped to the truck's floor and Tanya and I wrapped her in a sterile burn sheet. All the while, we asked, "where do you hurt, how bad is it?" Her answers helped us calculate the percent of her body surface burned, and to classify burns as first, second, or third-degree. We needed to determine if her airway or critical areas were burned. Uncomfortable pain might mean first-degree; screaming pain second-degree; no pain in a burned area meant third-degree.

"I can't leave my son! I'm OK!"

I said, "I promise we'll take good care of him. You have extensive burns, including your face, arms, and hands. This requires we get you to the burn center fast—meaning we will put you on a medevac helicopter."

She objected, "I'm a registered nurse. I don't need a helicopter; I'll go with you to the ER, but I must take care of my boy. Can you call my mother?"

Tanya telephoned the 911-dispatch center and repeated the phone number the patient gave us to reach her mother. Tanya used the telephone, not the radio. We didn't broadcast personal information over open radio waves.

The firefighter-driver lit the lights and siren and headed out as we continued our treatments.

I said to Tanya, "Partner, I'm starting two IVs, so please put together two saline drip sets."

Because the patient was a nurse, I used technical explanations and elaborated the details of what we were doing and why. I wanted to establish rapport and get her to focus on us and on the information we needed from her.

"Maam, I'll give you a dose of Zofran to prevent nausea, then morphine to help with the pain. We'll be infusing two bags of normal saline fast, so we must use large-bore needles. We'll only waste time by going to the ER. They'll have to fly you to the burn center once they see you. You burned your face, your airway might be injured, and you certainly have damage to your elbow, wrist, and hand joints. Burn scars around those joints could cripple you for life. The helicopter crew will include a flight nurse and a paramedic."

She nodded, the first sign of calming. Then she told us what had happened. "I was preparing a relaxing bath for myself. I filled the tub with water, put my son on the floor in his chair. I struck a match to light candles, and the bathroom just blew up! Oh my God, there was a blinding flash and fire. Are you sure he's all right?"

"Yes, he is. We called your mother, and she's on her way to get him. Police and EMS are taking care of him until she arrives. Dispatch confirmed another paramedic checked out your son, and he's uninjured."

As I examined her face, it morphed into my sister's. Was it my sister screaming, her arms outstretched in front of her? Or was it the siren? I startled, shook my head, and the face became my patient's once again.

"You OK?" Tanya whispered, her eyes narrowing.

I nodded.

The driver didn't throw us around. He was experienced and knew to use all the different siren yelps and frequent air horn blasts to warn other drivers, and to protect us by turning and braking carefully.

I started two large-bore IVs, one in each arm, aiming for the biggest veins I could see in her forearms. We usually tried for the antecubital space, the bend in the front of an elbow where big veins are easiest. But with her burns, I wanted to avoid the joints so as not to endanger treatments or healing. Fluid loss can quickly lead to death in burn patients, and the body shunts all the fluids it can to burned areas. I adjusted the drip rates to wide-open. By the time the medevac helicopter flew the seventy miles to the burn center, she would get at least two liters of saline for fluid replacement.

We arrived at the landing zone where the medevac chopper was already on the ground and waiting to transfer the patient from our unit. The flight crew clambered into our unit to get my report and do an initial patient assessment. That done, firefighters rushed the stretcher out to the waiting bird. The chopper lifted off within seconds of securing the stretcher onboard.

With the patient now in expert hands, I sagged on the rear bumper of our unit, cradled my head in my hands, my elbows on my knees, my legs turned to rubber, and stared at the ground. Keying my radio, I said, "County, Unit Five will be out of service until further notice."

Tanya sagged next to me, both of us drained, our reserves of energy empty. It was the adrenalin and concern that drained us, not the physical work we had done.

Ordinarily, only a supervisor would take a unit out of service. A crew chief could do this in extraordinary circumstances, if he or she believed it essential. I deemed it essential.

Our captain came to our station the next day to tell us what happened. "A natural gas pipe ran under her house to the neighbor's house behind hers. The old pipe rusted and sprang leaks, releasing gas, which the neighbor smelled in his house. The gas company repaired the line on his property. They shut the gas off in his yard to make the repairs, damming the gas flow, which increased pressure in the line in her yard, causing gas to seep into her bathroom. When she lit a match, she sparked a flash fireball. Luckily, it only damaged her bathroom, and only from knee-high to the ceiling. Gas is lighter than air, so it filled the room from the ceiling down. Her son, sitting on the floor and below the tub's rim, escaped injury.

"By the way, Sarge, that woman is an old friend of mine. I called to see how she's doing at the burn center. She told me you wouldn't listen to her when she said she didn't need to go there. Well, she heard today she'll be there quite a while for skin grafts and therapy. She's lucky she's there. You did well. What made you think she needed the burn center when as a nurse she didn't think so?"

"Honestly, the way she was sitting on the steps holding her arms out, like a little girl reaching for her mother."

Tanya said, "I guess you saw zebras."

"I've never lost a patient because of noticing details. I've always found a big part of getting the right diagnosis and treatment plan is not getting the wrong diagnosis. And when I hear hoofbeats, I ask do they really mean zebras? The safest strategy is to assume they might."

Tanya said, "Your sister saved that woman."

The nurse who argued she didn't need a helicopter spent two weeks in the burn center. She walked out without complications or disfiguring scars.

Most paramedics would have accepted her objections as coming from an expert, a registered nurse, who knew what she was talking about. They would have taken her to the ER, as she insisted, or waited around at the scene until her mother arrived to take her son. On the scene, the burns might have looked minor. Other paramedics might hear hoofbeats and see the horses they expected to see.

Now, I can no longer live like other people. Like people who are always looking at their phones and not the world around them, not watching for the zebra stampede, or the car trying to beat the yellow light, or painful red skin and arms stretched out. You can leave EMS, but EMS never leaves you. Not totally.

Because I noticed details and looked for zebras, she lives with full mobility.

Seven years later, I still see her with crystal clarity, sitting on the front steps, arms outstretched, frantic, crying out. I see her blue bathrobe and and smell curling wisps of acrid smoke.

But now, four years after retiring, I imagine her screams instead of hearing them.

2010- Her First Day In Daycare

She died.

No one knew when or why.

The daycare owner, Margaret, had been holding the infant, walking and soothing her with gentle bounces against a matronly chest, humming quietly. Another child squealed and Margaret laid the two-month-old on the sofa. Then Margaret turned her attention to care for the other child's needs.

The owner finished with the other child and turned back to the infant. The tiny angel appeared to sleep. But something had changed. She lay too still.

Bobby and I walked into the substation after our twelve-hour shift started with three early calls in a row. We shared one station computer to write reports.

"Bobby, I'm going to finish my call report; it'll take just five minutes more. Then, the computer is yours."

"Okay Sarge. I'll wash my hands while you finish up."

Bobby washed his hands before and after every call, and after each station duty. He was as conscientious as a surgeon about hand washing. I considered Bobby one of the best EMT-Intermediates in the service. As dependable as the sun. Tanya was another great Intermediate, and these two were my favorite partners. With the chief's policy of rotating partners, I only worked with one or the other maybe twice a month.

The quiet was splintered by the radios hooked to our shoulder epaulets, "Unit-Four, County, emergency traffic."

Keying my mic, I said, "County, Unit-Four on our way." We headed back out to the dripping wet ambulance.

"Partner, you drive," I said, heading toward the passenger side.

"You got it, Saaarge," he drawled in his best John Wayne imitation. This was our fourth call in as many hours and meant we would go home more exhausted than usual.

Bobby started the engine and lit up the emergency lights as I unhooked the dashboard radio, stretched the cord and thumbed the radio switch, "County, Unit-Four responding."

"Unit-Four, County, pediatric arrest."

Pediatric Arrest! A child dead. The second of my most dreaded calls.

In the adjoining fire station lights flickered, followed by alarm tones, and then dispatch broadcast over the public address system: "Engine four, pediatric arrest."

Bobby's jaw muscles bunched as he clenched his teeth. Ordinarily, he pulled out of a station as carefully as a stretch limo chauffeur. This time, he launched us from the driveway, acceleration pinning me into the seatback. This was one of his nightmare calls too.

An ambulance driver can't see well to the right because a big GPS/computer display mounted between us blocked his view. Vision to the rear didn't exist with the boxy patient compartment behind the cab. Bobby watched traffic on the left and ahead. I watched to the right, and tracked our progress on the GPS screen.

"Bobby, when we get there, you bring the jump bag into the house, fast. Don't bother with the gurney. Leave that to the firefighters. I'm going straight into the daycare!"

Bobby responded, "Got it."

It was only a few minutes until we arrived on scene. We rounded a curve on a long, tree-lined driveway, and a surreal scene greeted us. A white, professionally made sign on a small, well-groomed front lawn proclaimed it a daycare center. A two-story house sat in a clearing at the edge of woods. It was a Victorian confection with fish-scale shingles, a turret, and wrap-around porches all painted white and blue. A glossy wood door with a view window stood open at the top of a raised front porch. This whole scene struck me as charming, a puzzling reaction given the nature of this call.

As Bobby skidded to a stop, I forced myself back into the moment, leaped from the unit, bolted up the porch stairs three at a time, and rushed into a large living room. A decorated Christmas tree with its twinkling lights stood against one wall.

Margaret, the only adult present, pointed toward the sofa, saying, "It's her first day in daycare."

The tiny infant looked so peaceful, so angelic, with only the slightest hint of bluish-gray, more an impression than a color.

I will not let Death take my patient! Snatching her up, her body was loose and floppy with the total limpness of death. I struggled to stay composed, in control. If I lost it, there would be no one to help her right now when she needed help. I had to focus on the mechanics, on what to do now. Then on what to do next.

I put my ear to her face. I so desperately wanted to hear a breath, to prove the daycare owner and the 911 dispatcher were wrong. Infant cardiac arrest usually stems from a breathing problem, so my first step was to try rescue breaths.

I broke the cardinal rule of BSI—Body Substance Isolation—instantly tilting her head back to open her airway. Covering the tiny bluish mouth and nose with my lips, I blew twice into her, just hard enough to begin a slight rise in her chest. It's too easy to burst an infant's lungs with adult breaths. Her chest didn't move, and her saliva blew back into my mouth.

Shit! A nanosecond of horror gripped me: I had been exposed to body fluids!

I went back to work, readjusted her head by tilting it backward a bit more, and breathed for her again. Her little chest rose a fraction of an inch as air entered her lungs.

I had gained precious seconds by rushing from the ambulance without grabbing equipment. But I lost the safety provided by the rescue face mask carried in the jump bags.

Two more breaths followed by two-finger chest compressions. The two-finger technique uses the index and middle fingers on the baby's sternum, pointing straight at the heart, and looks like a deep and forceful poking of the chest.

I counted to fifteen before stopping for two more rescue breaths—the cycle I repeated until Bobby could take over breathing for her.

Bobby ran in and without a word snatched a baby-sized oxygen mask from the jump bag. He took over bag-valve-mask ventilations, and my anxiety eased with him beside me. He's a pro and didn't hesitate even a fraction of a second. I repositioned my hands, thumb-to-thumb on her sternum, the standard position for two-person infant cardiac CPR. Because her body was so tiny, I had to overlap my fingers around her torso.

We worked with only the count of compressions spoken aloud. This kept us focused and alert to upcoming pauses for him to squeeze the Ambu-bag ventilator.

The roar of a fire truck's diesel engine and the squeal of heavy-duty brakes carried through the open front door. Two firefighters rushed in. One said, "Jake is at the ambulance. He'll be your driver." These guys knew exactly what was needed, and they did not waste a second asking for instructions.

Holding the baby's lifeless body, we double-timed from the house. With the infant cradled in the crook of my left arm, I switched to two-finger compressions. Bobby matched me step for step as he squeezed the ventilation bag and held the mask tight to her face. We laid her on the stretcher in the ambulance, a fireman closed the doors, and I called out, "Let's go!"

The trip to the ER is a jumbled blur of images and sounds:

...Bobby and I moving together seamlessly in what would look frenzied to an outsider.

...Bobby inserting an infant airway into her mouth.

...Me attaching miniature cardiac leads to her chest.

...One hundred percent oxygen flowing full open.

...Bobby squeezing the smallest Ambu-bag we carried.

...Both of us watching the cardiac monitor for blood-oxygen content and for a change from a flat line to a heartbeat.

...Both of us trying to will her little heart into beating again.

...Counting seconds aloud between respirations.

...calling out the count of compressions and breaths.

The noise in the rig was deafening as we screamed down the highway, sirens and air horn blasting, the diesel motor roaring.

I yelled over the din to the driver, "Get on the radio, call the ER, warn them what's going on, and give them an ETA!" Pausing CPR to do my radio report was not an option.

Emergency room staff started preparations as we sped to get there. An anesthesiologist stood by to insert a tube into the trachea. A respiratory therapist brought in a ventilation machine to take over breathing. One nurse prepared to continue chest compressions, another readied IVs. Yet another got the drug cart in place, One more prepared to log actions and times. And the primary ER doc stood like the conductor in front of an orchestra, ready to set the tempo and lead the life-saving symphony of action. Fourteen pairs of hands compared to mine and Bobby's four.

My partner and I in the lurching ambulance doing the only thing we could—manual CPR. We could only breathe for her, pump her blood for her. We dare not stop to start an IV or prepare drugs.

Our EMS supervisor, a captain, met us as we pulled into the ER parking bay. She asked, "Any change, any pulse?"

"No," The only reply I could manage.

The captain and the firefighter-driver took charge of pushing the stretcher with the infant on it. Bobby hurried alongside on the gurney's left side, I was on the right. We never stopped chest compressions or ventilations. We swung into the room waiting for us; the room packed with fourteen pairs of hands all intent on saving this baby.

I had to shout my report to the lead physician to be heard over the nurses. They scrambled to help us, calling instructions to each other and reports to the doctor. The baby disappeared in a phalanx of nurses, doctors, and technicians.

I pushed myself into a corner, watching the scene with fading hope. The monitor mounted near the ceiling showed the dreaded flat green line. The physicians and nurses worked hard to restart her heart, but then the doctor said, "time of death..."

The doctor beckoned the parents to come in, allowing them to say goodbye to their baby. The daycare operator must have phoned them. How else could they be here? Stepping out to the nurse's station, I swiped at a tear in the corner of my eye, choked down a sob, and nodded thanks to the nurse who placed a hand on my shoulder.

Turning to my captain, I mumbled, "There's a complication. I gave mouth-to-mouth to the baby, and I got her spit in my mouth. I didn't take time to grab a face mask."

The captain shut her eyes and her shoulders slumped. Then, she took my arm and guided Bobby and me out to the EMS waiting room.

She closed the door then said, "Oh, you didn't! Damn it! I understand why, it was a baby, but you know better. Remember Sebastian, the Florida deputy? He died last week after giving mouth-to-mouth to a three-month-old who had meningitis."

"Yes, I read about him in the safety bulletin. Sorry, Captain." My apology was the correct thing to say and likely sounded contrite. But I only felt drained, not contrite.

The Captain said, "We've got to report this. Go to the County services unit and fill out the necessary paperwork. They'll coordinate any treatment for you with the ER here. You know I'll need your written statement about the exposure incident today. Before you go home! No questions. And Bobby, I'll need a report from you too. Damn it!"

The County took exposures seriously. There was sure to be a reprimand in my file in the coming days. There would be blood tests on both the baby and me for HIV, hepatitis, TB, meningitis, and sexually transmitted infections.

"Unit-Four, County, emergency call holding." My radio thundered into our little group meeting.

We were the closest unit to a call too urgent to wait for a more distant ambulance. The dispatcher wouldn't know we had lost the baby.

Lying to myself and my captain, I said, "I'm OK. We have a call waiting."

And Bobby and I headed for our unit in the parking bay to respond to yet another 911 call for help.

We were the people who did CPR on a baby by the light of a Christmas tree, all the while knowing deep down what we didn't want to know. Because we were there, Margaret had hope in her eyes. She didn't know what lay ahead, but we did.

In the following days, I brooded over this call. What was the worst part? Was it the tiny infant dying; or watching the parents say goodbye; or how I went home broken-hearted, kissed my wife assuring her it was just another day? I still don't know.

I straddled a fence about this call. The infant died before I got to her. But that did not change the terrible, breath-stealing sadness because I couldn't bring her back. When I was nine, I vowed I would beat Death. But I meant I would prevent a death; I didn't mean I would perform a resurrection.

I told myself I had not lost this baby girl, that she was gone before I got to her. I told myself over and over.

I redoubled my efforts to beat Death every chance I got.

2011- And the Ground Opened Up

It was a quiet day, the early Fall weather nice, and we'd had only one 911 call so far this shift. I was the crew chief and paramedic on Unit-Five, sitting in our eight-by-ten EMS station which shared walls with the fire department. Bobby, my partner today, read a hunting magazine while I did paperwork on the desktop computer. Bobby was a quiet one, always watching and listening, but he could cut up with a practical joke among friends. He appeared shy and lacking confidence until you got to know him. When it came to emergency medicine on the street, he was smart as a whip and hard as a telephone pole.

"Unit-Five, County, Emergency traffic, fire standby."

Fire standby meant we were going as a medical backup to fire-crews, usually already on some sort of call that 911 dispatch did not at first think needed an ambulance. Maybe the initial call was a minor fender-bender that turned into something more complicated. Perhaps it was a small brush fire, or a kitten stuck in a tree. But something changed, and now an ambulance should be on the scene, just in case, or to do periodic checks on the condition of firefighters. But we could also be dispatched at the same time as the fire crews. Structure fires always meant a fire-standby call out, these calls being inherently more dangerous.

Bobby keyed his radio mike, "County, Unit-Five is responding."

We stood and headed to our ambulance, which sat at the curb in front of our door. Just then, the air filled with the urgent screams of multiple fire engine sirens and the roar of their big diesel engines starting up only twenty yards from us.

Uh Oh!

We climbed into the ambulance and, with emergency lights strobing and siren whooping, headed toward the neighborhood showing on our GPS computer. It looked like it was less than a mile away. The big hook-and-ladder pulled out of the fire station right behind us, followed by the remaining two fire trucks and the fire captain's SUV. Every available truck and man at this station was rolling. Bobby and I were leading a charging single-file parade of responding emergency vehicles, all going to the same place, which surely was not a fender-bender.

In less than a minute, we pulled into a cul-de-sac in a residential neighborhood. My partner parked our ambulance three houses short of the address, leaving room for the fire engines to pull up in front of the actual scene. We expected carnage or smoke or bodies. But there was no smoke, no crumpled vehicles, no bodies lying on the ground. There was only an older gentleman a few feet from our ambulance, holding a small dog to his chest, bent at the waist and staring at the grass between his feet.

"What's going on Bobby?"

"Don't know Sarge."

I stepped out and walked up to the gentleman asking, "Sir, can we help you?"

I heard Bobby's radio transmission to Dispatch, "County, Unit-Five is on scene."

Up close, I could see he wasn't staring at the grass, but at a dark, round hole in the ground. It was only about nineteen inches in diameter, maybe even less than that.

"Help," the older gentleman cried.

"My wife is stuck down there."

That's when we heard a muffled, "Help me please! I'm stuck and sliding down!"

The fire chief in charge overheard this exchange and immediately started issuing orders and instructions to all his firefighters.

A firefighter ran to a truck to get a length of rope; several others quick-marched to the big ladder engine, grabbing metal pipes, and began to set up a tripod over the hole. They attached a pulley to the top of this and prepared to feed the rope through it. There wasn't a single storage cabinet on the side of any fire truck that wasn't clanged open to give immediate access to equipment.

The fire chief asked the older gentleman, "What happened? How did she get into this hole?"

"I was out walking our dog. We always walk along this stretch of grass for him to do his business. Suddenly the ground opened up under him, and he fell into the hole. I couldn't reach him, so I yelled for my wife to come help. She came running from our front yard, and she reached down while I held her. She got the dog up, but when I let go of her to grab the dog from her, she just somehow slipped or lost her balance and fell into the hole."

The woman was at least four feet down. She called up to us that she wasn't injured, but nobody had any idea how deep this old well might be. I later learned some wells went down a mere sixty feet, and some were a few hundred feet deep. She was in grave peril, even if she didn't fall any further. She could suffocate right where she was or succumb to hypothermia. Besides a rescue rope, we needed to run tubing down to her to supply oxygen. Air doesn't circulate more than a couple of feet down into narrow holes.

The fire chief started asking all of us for ideas. Could she hold on to the rope with enough strength while being pulled up? Probably not. Could she tie the rope around herself? No, she couldn't move her arms enough to do that. Could we lower the smallest firefighter down to her? Maybe, if wearing no gear, but he'd have to go down headfirst. Can we dig around the well-hole to get more access? We don't know what equipment is needed or how available it is.

After a quarter-hour of brain storming, all the while talking confidently to the woman to assure her help was here, my EMS captain advised us to head back to our station to handle more immediate emergency calls. We had no idea how long this rescue would take. He was on scene and would radio for an ambulance if needed.

The captain never called for a unit, so we knew the patient was okay, and apparently did not need an ambulance. We never found out more details of the story of how she came to fall into that well. Both fire and EMS crews speculated wildly.

She fell in feet first. Once the dog was up, did she then step into the hole herself? Did she really slip, or did the older-gentleman-holding-the-little-dog-to-his-chest-husband help her in? That last was just our version of gallows humor, not serious. But we never got the answer.

What we learned is there are hundreds of old wells like this in the county. They were supposed to be sealed with permanent caps, but too often some farmer did nothing more than place a half-sheet of three-quarter-inch plywood over the old well and covered it with soil. That method guaranteed the well cover was temporary, lasting only until the plywood rotted away. If the soil was covered with decorative sod, as in newer, pleasant neighborhoods like this was, then it was a potential trapdoor leading to a terrible death by suffocation.

2012- The Golden Hour

There is a concept in emergency medicine: the Golden Hour. After a traumatic injury, the patient's best odds of surviving are if he or she can get to a trauma surgeon within one hour.

There is a related idea: the **Platinum Ten Minutes**. The idea is the ambulance crew starts transport to the ER within ten minutes of arriving on the scene.

In a small county such as where I work, an event might look like this. After a life-threatening injury, it could take five minutes for someone to dial 911; four minutes to dispatch the unit; seven minutes for the ambulance to get to the scene; ten minutes on scene while the crew stops serious bleeding and ensures patient breathing, loads the patient into the ambulance, and starts for the ER; with no traffic delays, that trip might average twenty minutes. Time elapsed before seeing the trauma specialist: forty-six minutes. Leaving a doctor a scant fourteen minutes inside that golden hour. Every minute past the Platinum-ten on scene robs the doctor's time, robs the patient's chances.

Time management is critical in our line of work, and the only periods I control are how fast we get the wheels rolling after being toned out, and the time spent on scene.

The two-way radio shattered the silence in the EMS station, "Unit 4, County, emergency traffic."

Tanya and I were relaxing back in our substation after a call and run to the ER. We were now on the western edge of the county.

I responded, "County, Unit Four en route to the truck."

With the radio alert the adrenalin rush started and my heart rate rose from my average fifty beats per minute. Another call from Dispatch, another life possibly in the balance. We couldn't know until we arrived on the scene.

Tanya started the motor as I slid into the passenger seat. Keying the radio, she said, "County, Unit Four responding."

Radio transmissions were brief. In four words Tanya got the attention of who she was talking to, identified our unit, and that we were in the ambulance and ready to roll.

"Unit Four, County, hemorrhage at..." and the dispatcher announced the address. It looked like three miles, maybe four minutes, through the center of this small town.

I said, "Damn, why do they always call it hemorrhage? Why don't they just say nosebleed? In four years of hemorrhage calls, that's all I've ever found—a nosebleed. I can't recall when a nose still bled by the time we arrived."

Tanya said, "I know what you mean. We don't want somebody dying, but why call for an ambulance when it will stop in ten more minutes on its own? We don't swat mosquitoes with hammers, do we?"

We pulled into the roadway with emergency lights flashing and siren wailing. In the center of town Tanya turned left, and in seconds we drove along a two-lane residential street heading toward the address Dispatch gave us.

Two blocks ahead a woman was frantically waving her arms and jumping up and down, her ponytail bouncing. I said, "There, on the right, see that lady doing jumping jacks to wave us down? This doesn't look good!"

I put on my disposable gloves and laid my partner's on the center console. Tanya braked and I jumped down, hurrying toward the distraught woman as Tanya radioed Dispatch that we had arrived on scene.

Walk, don't run, stay calm, and take control of the situation. BSI—body substance isolation—scene safe; the mantra drummed into every EMT.

As I approached, the woman bolted toward her front door, yelling, "He's in here! This way!"

This isn't a typical nosebleed. Striding through the front door, I did a quick scan of the room, as I had a half second to make sure no dangers lurked inside and to assess the urgency of the situation.

A middle-aged man sat on a straight-backed kitchen chair in the living room.

He looked calm and fit, except for the towel he held against his neck. Blood poured from between his fingers. Sweat beaded on his pale forehead. He didn't move or say a word. Silent, pale, still and calm. Still and calm were reassuring signs. Pale wasn't. He stared up at me with frightened eyes.

Shock hit me instantly, like getting ice water in the face. I couldn't breathe, couldn't think, couldn't even move. Then I snapped to and rushed forward.

It looks like this guy's bleeding out! Is it jugular or carotid or both?

I focused on the job at hand. I learned long ago dangerous things were worth being afraid of. But I had beat Death before, and battles I had won did not justify fear. To be afraid of a winnable situation was irrational. I was a rational man. *I am a paramedic, and I will beat Death again.*

I replaced his hand with my gloved hand, keeping direct pressure on.

Blood ran between my fingers and puddled on the floor. A lake of blood was spreading around my boots.

My heart hammered like a rapid drum roll in my chest.

"What happened?" I asked.

It was the woman who answered. "He just got home from the hospital where he had a stent placed in his carotid artery."

His lips quivered and blood bubbled from his mouth, flowing down his chin. His frightened eyes said, "Don't let me die."

His life was spurting out of him—a severed carotid artery emptying itself too fast. His heart was doing its job, pumping rapidly, but now it was pumping his life away.

Tanya hurried into the room, and without a second's hesitation or a single word, opened the 75-pound jump bag she had carried in, tore open a large absorbent sterile pad, and handed it to me.

I told her, "It's hard to tell how much blood he's lost, but I estimate at least half-a-liter. He had a carotid stent placed this morning. He's bleeding into his airway as well as externally. Lean him forward and let the blood flow out and not down his throat."

I strained to keep my voice calm and collected. Blood irritates the stomach and retching or vomiting now would jerk his throat from my hand. That would be fatal.

I lifted the blood-soaked towel to replace it with the sterile pressure dressing. A pulse of blood spurted across the room, spraying the wall—*open carotid artery!*

I applied as much pressure as possible while avoiding his trachea. I needed to stop the bleeding, not his breathing. We pushed him forward from the waist to let the blood drain from his mouth.

Nobody taught us how to treat a slit throat or ruptured carotid artery. They figured by the time we arrived a patient would be beyond treatment. Dozens of aphorisms abound in EMS to cement lessons in our minds. One is: *Don't panic; all bleeding ends eventually.* Yes, when the patient bleeds out.

And that's what my patient was doing, sitting in his living room, his carotid artery spurting both down his throat and out onto the carpet! It wasn't the platinum ten minutes—it was a life or death ten seconds.

Critical decisions were needed: how to get him into the ambulance? How to get an emergency driver? Which of two routes to the ER?

We no longer had the Platinum ten minutes. Tanya had pushed the stretcher from the ambulance to the front steps. She could not get it up the stairs and into the house by herself.

Normally, I plan by talking to myself. Now, I thought in flashes of images, like a movie at double fast speed. I pictured Tanya supporting the patient; me holding pressure; us walking down the front steps to the stretcher; Tanya calling ahead for a firefighter to meet us along the route to the ER. We would pass four fire stations driving through towns, each being a chance to get a driver on board. We would not be able to get a driver if we took the interstate.

I hit the mental "Play" button and put us in motion.

"Tanya, we are going to walk him between us to the gurney, then you will have to push it while I maintain pressure. You will drive through town and radio ahead for an emergency driver. Keep driving and calling until we get one."

We quick-marched the patient to the gurney outside.

Once we made it inside the ambulance, Tanya ran around to the driver's seat and hit siren, lights, and gas all at once. I stretched for the handset left-handed, my right hand pressing on the dressing against the side of his neck.

"County ER, Unit Four, emergency traffic!" I barked out the last two words. I needed a nurse or doctor on their radio immediately. And I wanted all other units to clear the airway and give us priority. We all used the same radio channel.

"Unit Four, County ER, go ahead."

"County ER, Unit Four is inbound, emergent, with a carotid artery hemorrhage following surgical complication. Bleeding is external and internal into the airway. I'm maintaining manual pressure and trying to keep his airway clear by sitting position. Patient's alert and oriented, no other vitals possible. ETA 20 minutes. Unit Four clear."

"Unit Four, County ER, copy. Report any changes. County ER standing by."

I marveled at the nurse's calm tone. They train nurses to remain calm on radio calls. Usually though, some emotion came across. Not this time. What I did hear was the unsaid meaning of "Report any changes." What she was telling me was to radio ahead if I lost him, if I pronounced him dead en route.

Tanya shouted through the pass-through opening from the cab to the patient compartment, "We're coming up on the first meeting point near the first station. I see the fire truck parked in the center lane."

I yelled to be heard over the engine and siren, "Stop behind them, jump out and get back here!"

Tanya climbed through the back doors only seconds after throwing the transmission into Park. The firefighter-now-driver called out from the driver's seat, "Where to?"

I replied, "County ER, and make it fast but smooth. Don't throw us around!" If I bounced away from the gurney, if I lost hand pressure against his neck, the patient could die.

They train paramedics to always instill confidence in patients and families by displaying calmness. Among ourselves, we joked this was the duck technique: look calm on the surface and don't let them see you are paddling like hell below.

We work fast and we're not dainty on an ambulance, because many people who are able to make it through the Golden Hour just can't make it for one minute more. Tanya was opening sterile, absorbent dressings as fast as what I held soaked through. We never replaced sterile dressings that controlled bleeding, we added to them. Removing a dressing would dislodge a forming blood clot that should stem the bleeding.

She was also taking frequent blood pressure and heart rate readings, intent on spotting impending, irreversible shock.

My self-control was at the red line. I literally held his life in my hands. I strained to keep him off the list of those I lost, which so far stood at zero.

The patient remained eerily calm, although his eyes pleaded with Tanya and me.

When he tried to mumble, Tanya said, "Don't talk! Just keep spitting the blood out as best you can." He did, and turned the cot and floor into a blood bath.

The firefighter blasted the air horn as he slalomed through intersections and traffic.

Tanya called out, "Sarge, his pressure is at ninety systolic, dropping slowly, and his heart rate is okay at one-thirty-five."

A systolic pressure below one hundred called for me to start an IV and push normal saline to help his heart. But I needed four arms to do that. It was not an option now.

The driver turned into the ER drive. An emergency room nurse waited for us in the parking bay. They only did this in dire situations. The driver and Tanya were pulling the gurney out while I started the climb from the unit. The nurse put one hand in the small of my back as I stepped down the three-and-a-half feet from the ambulance floor to the driveway. I prayed I wouldn't fall and release the pressure on his neck.

We rushed the gurney through sliding emergency department doors, leaving a trail of bloody footprints. We turned a corner and standing there were a trauma surgeon and five RNs, all dressed in surgical gowns and plastic face shields. They had prepared for arterial spray should the patient still be alive. The team gathered around the stretcher, and eight pairs of hands lifted the patient onto a bed as I kept manual pressure on his neck.

I gave the doctor my report, "Carotid stent placed this morning, left side. Bleeding started minutes after arriving at home, and it's both external and internal. Based on systolic pressure of ninety and dropping, and heart rate at one-thirty-five, I estimate one-third volume lost, the patient's still in compensated shock."

The doctor took over direct pressure from me, eased the pressure dressing corner, and said: "Good job, now we'll get this repaired. Nurse, order two units of blood, and let the bank know he was operated on this morning. They'll have his blood-type information." The doctor seemed as calm and resolute as granite.

Tanya, the firefighter-driver, and I left the room as a nurse pulled the window drapes and closed the door. They were about to do emergency surgery right there.

We walked to the EMTs' waiting room and collapsed onto hard chairs. Other EMT crews taking breaks between calls volunteered to clean the the blood and debris from the back of our truck, which now looked like a MASH unit in a combat zone. Every crew in the county heard my radio transmission to the ER.

Tanya and I changed our blood-soaked uniforms before leaving the hospital. County policy dictated each crew member carry a spare change of uniform in our personal duty duffels, which we stowed in crew storage compartments on the ambulance.

We had done our duty, lived up to our calling, and learned days later the patient was home and doing well. My count remained at zero. I would never again stereotype a tone-out. Not for a hemorrhage—not for anything.

I celebrated beating Death once again. I felt good, even cocky.

2013-Santa Claus

The following month, Tanya and I were back sitting in substation four, on the western edge of the county. Besides being the paramedic on this ambulance, I was the crew chief, the one in charge, the one responsible. I considered it the best job in the service. I had a job to do, but I got to do it my way. To be designated as a crew chief we had to impress our superiors during a four-week training period after graduating paramedic school. We had to prove we made efficient decisions under pressure. The training officer emphasized efficient as both effective and quick.

Tanya and I had finished our reports for the first two calls of this shift.

"So, Papa, the first time you did CPR happened in a bank. When was that?"

I had just finished telling her the story about the old man in the California bank and my first time doing CPR. She sat in a recliner an arm's length away in this one-room station.

"Tanya, that was 1983, a quarter-century ago. Before you were out of grade school."

"Well Sarge, you are an old man." She tossed her head, swinging strands of shoulder-length hair out of her face, and tried to suppress a giggle, but failed.

"Hey girl, just because nobody remembers another codger starting paramedic school in his sixties doesn't make me an old man. Ten years later, I still outrun the young whipper-snappers around here."

She laughed. "Yeah, you're right. I don't see anyone else keeping up with you. You go back a long way."

"I go back so damn far it isn't funny."

Tanya was a Southern girl, as comfortable on a horse ranch as in a ballroom. Middle age was still over the horizon for her. She was heading toward forty years younger than me. Not tall, maybe an inch or two over average for women. She radiated a vitality that took the word medium out of the picture. She was halfway between curvy and athletic. Her hair was short and fair.

"Unit Four, County, emergency traffic," our radios interrupted our storytelling. We stood in unison.

We each had a radio microphone attached to our shoulder epaulets, with a spiral elastic cord stretched down to the radio hooked to our duty belts. Tanya reached up to her shoulder and pressed the transmit button on the mic, "County, Unit Four en route." En route meant we were heading toward our ambulance.

With stethoscopes draped around our necks, we only needed to grab our jackets as we hustled to the ambulance parked in the bay. Tanya climbed into the driver's seat as I went around the truck's hood to the passenger side. She started the engine and switched on emergency lights and sirens.

I keyed the dashboard radio, "County, Unit Four responding." Responding—meaning we were in our ambulance and ready to roll after Dispatch gave us the address and the call's details.

"Unit Four, County, unconscious male, possible cardiac arrest at..." They confirmed the address that appeared on the computer screen.

Tanya pulled onto the street as traffic stopped in both directions. "OK partner," I said, "I'll go in with the cardiac monitor; you bring the jump bag. We'll leave the stretcher for the fire crew to bring in. Let's hope they are on scene or right behind us."

Tanya didn't need a gentleman to carry the seventy-five pound jump bag crammed with enough supplies to strain the canvas seams. She looked soft and curved in the right places, but was strong enough to run with the best while carrying the jump bag. I needed an EKG on the scene, immediately, so I would carry the thirty-pound portable cardiac monitor.

Dispatch always toned a fire truck out to a call for an unconscious patient or reported cardiac arrest. Fire crews used the term *toned*, referring to the initial loud emergency signal using the fire station's klaxon horn. This alerted fire crews to listen for their emergency message over the PA (public address) system. In EMS, we used electronic *tones* on our radios preceding a dispatcher's message, like a weather alert. This signaled the specific crew receiving the tone to pay attention, they were about to get an emergency message.

Firefighters helped us carry equipment, lift patients, and, if needed, drive the ambulance to the ER. Having a driver meant my partner stayed with me to help treat the patient. If firefighters arrived at the scene before us, they could provide oxygen, check for breathing and pulses, and start CPR if needed. They proved invaluable, especially a three- or four-man crew. Maybe once a year a lone volunteer firefighter was our only backup. When only one came, we swallowed hard, adapted, and improvised.

We pulled up at a double-wide mobile home. A fire truck which had followed us parked beside our ambulance. Tanya and I grabbed our equipment from the rear patient compartment, then strode to steps leading up to a narrow front door. Four firefighters climbed down from their engine and headed toward us.

Tanya called back to them, "Hey guys, can you get the stretcher and bring it up to these front steps? Thanks."

Two firefighters peeled off, heading to our unit. They opened the rear doors and took out the rolling gurney. The other two followed Tanya and me up the stairs. The stairs and front door were too narrow to get the gurney inside.

A middle-aged woman in a nightgown opened the door for us, then stepped back and began pacing in circles, crying, wringing her hands. A man only in underpants lay motionless on the living room floor. He looked to weigh at least 300 pounds, his neck so wide I was amazed anyone made shirts with collars that size. He sported a bushy white beard. He could have passed for Santa Claus.

I said, "He's unconscious, Tanya. If it was a simple fainting, he would have regained consciousness by now."

The wife said, "We... we were having, you know, sex... when he just grabbed his chest and fell right there."

"Tanya, please start oxygen." She was all business, grabbing the face mask and oxygen cylinder even as I spoke.

Placing two fingers on the left side of his neck, I bent with my ear to his nose and mouth, and looked down his chest. A rapid pulse quivered on my fingertips, and his belly rose with each breath.

"We've got a fast and thready pulse, and he's breathing. I'm getting an EKG." This alerted Tanya to pull back and not touch his body. I needed to see his heart beat, not a jumble of both of theirs.

Tanya called to the firefighters, "Bring in a spine board. We'll carry him on it to the gurney outside."

She was a great wingman. I attached three sticky EKG leads to his chest, Tanya pulled back, and we both watched the monitor's screen.

I said, "We have V-tach!"

Ventricular tachycardia, with the heart's chamber that pumped blood to the brain and body beating way too fast, over 250 beats per minute. The heart couldn't circulate life-saving blood at that rate. V-tach is a deadly rhythm. I needed to start an IV, administer Amiodarone, and radio to the ER doctor for orders to shock if that became necessary. This was the procedure according to our official treatment protocols.

We used Amiodarone as the first step in slowing a racing heartbeat. If Amiodarone didn't work, we got more aggressive and used cardioversion, what medics called shocking, or lighting up the patient. It's an electric shock strong enough to sometimes kill a helper if they're touching the patient. Shocking the patient meant stopping a patient's heart, a heart trying to pump. In essence, killing the patient, hopefully for just a few seconds. Also risking the lives of helpers or bystanders who might be collateral damage if they were touching the patient at the time of the shock. Being more risky, a doctor had to give us permission to do this maneuver.

Cardioversion can reboot the heart, something like a computer reboot. Unlike rebooting a computer by turning off it's electricity, we rebooted a heart by adding a jolt of electricity, a mini-electrocution. The heart stops beating for a few seconds, and the pause hopefully allows heart cells to calm down and synchronize into a regular rhythm.

I decided to move him from the house and into the ambulance. The service considered a scene as where the patient could be found. Seasoned paramedics operated by the dictum: *my scene is the patient compartment of the ambulance, a controlled environment with all my equipment. A controlled environment rolling toward the ER.*

"OK, guys, let's load and go."

Tanya said to the woman, "Ma'am, we need to get him to the ER. You can ride with us up front, or you can meet us at the County hospital—that's where we'll go."

"I'll ride with you. Oh my God!" She tied her nightgown shut and grabbed her purse from a coffee table.

I said, "We'll do everything we can, Ma'am."

I unplugged the EKG cord from the monitor, leaving the sticky leads attached to his chest.

The firefighters slid the long spine board under Santa with Tanya's help. As the firefighters lifted him, I hurried outside with the bulky monitor. Four firefighters cautiously tilted Santa through the door, then down the front steps, and onto the gurney. Now out of the house and on level ground, I put the monitor between his legs and plugged the chest leads back into the monitor. We took four rapid steps toward the ambulance when the monitor alarm sounded a full cardiac arrest. *Shit*! I had the presence of mind not to cuss aloud in front of his wife.

My chest seized tight with the hot flush of panic. The fear disappeared as suddenly as it had come. I focused on the job at hand. I was a paramedic, and I would beat Death.

"Let's go. We have an arrest!"

Tanya dropped the jump bag and immediately started chest compressions. One firefighter scooped up the bag and carried it while the others pushed the gurney. He lifted the bag into the ambulance, then ran around to the driver's seat. I carried the cardiac monitor through the side door into the back patient compartment. The firefighters pushed the gurney into the compartment through the rear double doors. The wheels folded up and the gurney slid inside. Tanya stopped chest compressions only for the two seconds it took for her and a firefighter to climb into the back. The firefighter immediately restarted compressions. Tanya took over ventilating the patient, and I prepared the electrodes to light the patient up. I didn't need a doctor's permission after the heart stopped in a cardiac arrest. There was nothing to lose, the patient was as good as dead.

The ride to the ER was frenzied activity. A firefighter stood and filled the narrow aisle next to the gurney doing chest compressions, his calves pushed against the bench seat, his knees against gurney. Tanya sat in the rear-facing captain's chair at the patient's head, squeezing the football-shaped Ambu-bag to breathe for him. I climbed over and around both of them to get equipment and drugs out of cabinets and drawers. Climbing into the narrow space between the firefighter and Tanya, I stretched the patient's left arm straight, clamping it between my knees so I could find a vein, start an IV, and push cardiac drugs.

The drugs didn't work. The green blip moving left to right on the monitor showed asystole, flat line, zero cardiac activity. I made a rushed radio report to the ER. Cardioversion was useless once a heart crashed to a flat line, leaving the only options—manual CPR, pushing drugs, and praying.

When we arrived at the hospital, we rushed the gurney into the ER. I raised my voice so the doctor could hear my report over the clamor as staff moved the patient from our gurney to an examination table. The roomful of nurses hustled about like a swarm of worker bees in a nest.

A nurse said to the doctor, "No response to epinephrine, no pulse, no blood pressure, asystole is continuous."

The doctor called out, "Time of death is..."

A heavy silence blanketed the room, and I turned and walked out.

I glimpsed the head nurse talking with Santa's wife, her head bowed, her hands covering her face, her shoulders shaking with sobs. At the nurses' station, all I could do was think through everything I had done, replaying the actions, looking for a missed opportunity, something—anything—that might have saved him.

A nurse touched my arm. "So you're the one who killed Santa Claus." It was her attempt at the ER version of gallows-humor. She thought I might laugh. Humor helps to fight off the tears that come with the job. It is somehow supposed to make reality a bit more tolerable. Our jokes were kept in private, and served as a coping mechanism to get us through the day.

All I could hear was a small voice inside my head saying, *you were wrong. Completely wrong.*

I had built my whole career on hearing it fewer times than the average medic. It was like a box score in my mind, and my score just plummeted. It upset me because I was a professional who was supposed to get things right, because to be wrong meant Death would win.

Santa was the first patient I lost after nine years as a paramedic. I couldn't wrap my mind around this. I did everything by the numbers, followed the treatment protocol to a T. But he died in my care. I'm not supposed to lose to Death when I do it right.

I thought, *Something's wrong.*

I was close to exhaustion, and mentally shattered. I had succeeded for fifty-plus years since not saving my sister, since vowing to beat Death, and it all fell apart in one terrible day. I did it by the book, but the patient died any way.

A week later, the lieutenant in charge of quality assurance critiqued my actions. She said, "I would have shocked him right there in the house. He was in unstable V-tach, dying, and he needed to be shocked."

I replied, "But the protocols say start an IV and give Amiodarone first, then call for orders to shock."

She said, "In my experience, that's what he needed, and that's what I would have done. You followed protocol so there won't be any repercussions. Just learn from this."

Learn? Learn what? That I could have lit Santa up and didn't because of a protocol? Learn I let Death win? Yeah, I learned lessons. First, Death won't be stopped just because I followed the rules. Second, thinking I could beat him might just be a lie. Following protocol was the proper thing to do, but it wasn't the right thing. What's the saying, it's better to ask forgiveness than permission?

The following year the County rewrote the V-tach orders. It gave us written permission to cardiovert first, before an IV and Amiodarone, in deadly heart rhythms like Santa's. The service considered me blameless for his death. But I still counted him as the first patient I killed. I could have lit Santa up, but didn't.

Finally, I had failed to beat Death, the first time since I was nine years old. I renewed my vow to not lose again.

2014- What Not to Do After A Gym Workout

"So, Papa, you've been quiet the last couple of months. Everything OK?"

Tanya and I were based at Station Five, on the outskirts of the County seat. This part of town was mixed residential and commercial. A rapid population growth added new businesses almost daily. Another gym had just opened, increasing the count to four within a three-mile radius.

"Yeah, I'm OK."

"You are not convincing me."

Tanya's Southern accent was more cultured than not, but you knew as a girl growing up she didn't shy away from football with the boys.

"I keep thinking about Santa. He's the first patient I ever lost. They warned us in paramedic class we would kill patients, and we had to prepare for that. We would make mistakes, not bring the right equipment with us, give the wrong drug, or give the right drug too late. They said we're only human, and if we couldn't deal with this, we had better quit the class right then and there. But I told myself not me. Yes, I might make mistakes, but never a fatal one."

"But you didn't make a mistake. You followed our standing orders."

"Yeah, I followed standing orders. But when Lieutenant Patti QA'd me, she said she would have immediately shocked. She's the best paramedic I know, and I feel guilty I didn't know what she knows."

Our training officer performed quality assurance reviews on every call where the patient died in our care or in the emergency room. It was assumed that if the patient died before being admitted to a room or surgery, our care might have been faulty.

"Come on, Papa, she's been at this for twenty years. You've been doing this what, seven?"

"No, nine years as a paramedic, eleven as an EMT. The Lieutenant was right; the old saying, it's better to ask for forgiveness than permission fit Santa's call to a T."

"Papa, you can't beat yourself up. You did nothing wrong. Think about what—the thousand you've saved? And, you've only lost one in nine years?" Tanya always made me smile when she called me *Papa*, her EMS Papa.

"Tanya, I don't know how many I saved, because that's not the count I keep. That's my job. I only count those I lose. Until Santa my count was zero."

Tanya replied, "Look Papa, normal medics don't get all depressed and down when they lose a patient."

I said, "Maybe they should."

Our radios interrupted, "Unit Five, County, emergency traffic."

Tanya responded, "County, Unit Five en route."

We grabbed our stethoscopes and headed for the ambulance. Tanya would drive; my tasks were to read the details sent from dispatch to our onboard computer, and to watch for traffic hazards on the right. With the driver's limited visibility to the right of the ambulance, we were trained to have the passenger call out "Clear Right" or "Traffic Right" to the driver. This became an automatic reflex habit for me, driving my wife crazy when riding with her in our car.

Once inside the ambulance, I keyed our radio, "County, Unit Five is responding."

The county tracked the time from when we received the alarm—the tone—to the time our truck's wheels started turning. They called this our response time. They held us to a sixty-second standard. In fact, real-time computer records tracked us from tone-out to arrival at the ER, and even how long we spent at the hospital before announcing we were back in service.

"Unit Five, County, male subject, trouble breathing..."

The dispatcher read out the address, confirming the information and GPS map route displayed on the computer. Emergency calls are like snow flakes, they seem to look the same, but each is unique. Novelty was a key benefit of this career.

Watching for traffic hazards to the right, I also made sure Tanya could see the GPS map by angling the screen more toward her. Traffic was cooperative, both directions pulling to their right, slowing, giving us the center lane. Tanya smiled and drawled, "Well, look at all these gentlemen, letting a lady go ahead."

I quipped, "A good lookin Lady."

She smiled, quickly and shyly, and kept on driving.

We pulled up to a tidy two-unit townhouse, and Tanya led the way as I carried our seventy-five pound medical jump bag. She knocked on the door, then stood aside to let her crew chief enter first to ensure the scene was safe. A Middle-Eastern woman in her early thirties opened the door. She was attractive in a native trouser and shirt outfit, even though she had a worried frown.

"My husband is here, on the floor behind the sofa. He cannot breathe." She spoke with a clipped accent.

Oh oh, on the floor isn't good. I hurried around her and behind the sofa. Being a hunter of trouble, I spotted it right away. The patient lay flat on his back, drenched with sweat, gulping great gasps of air, begging for breath like a fish out of water. His brow was lined with fear, his eyes pleading.

One look at the man told me we could not afford to spend time on scene. It was only a matter of minutes before he would be too fatigued to breathe.

I keyed my radio, "County, Unit Five, send fire emergent." The last three words communicated I needed several firefighters, and I needed them to run lights and sirens to get here fast. We needed the extra personnel to lift and move the patient rapidly, and one to drive so Tanya could stay with me and the patient in the rear compartment.

"Tanya, he's on the verge of respiratory arrest. Get oxygen set up and prepare for bagging if needed. This is a load-and-go."

Bagging meant using the silicon, football-shaped Ambu-bag to pump air into the patient's lungs. We carried four different sizes in the jump bag, ranging from baby to adult.

Tanya and I knelt on either side of him. I said, "Sir, can you tell me what happened when this started?"

I needed to test two things. First, was he alert and oriented, able to answer questions? Declining mental sharpness was the first sign of a slide toward death due to inadequate blood supply to the brain. Second, could he control his breathing well enough to talk?

"I just... got back... from the gym; I left because... I didn't feel well. When I got home... I started having... trouble getting... my breath. Now it's getting worse... harder to... breathe."

"Are you allergic to anything?"

"No."

"Are you taking any medications?"

"No... nothing."

"Do you have any medical conditions?"

"No... not... at all. I'm... only... thirty-two... and... healthy."

We watched his struggle to answer getting harder, so I stopped asking questions and sped up my actions. Tanya needed to get his vital signs. Grabbing a syringe, needle, and dressing from the jump bag, I started an IV in his arm while waiting for firefighters to arrive.

Tanya had trouble getting a good blood pressure reading and reported "Seventy palp, heart rate forty-six."

She had to palpate, feel the pulse in his wrist, because his blood pressure was too low to hear with her stethoscope. This only gave us half the normal reading, the systolic pressure, seventy in this case. Below one hundred, the lower limit we wanted to see. It was half the information we wanted, but the best she could do. And, a heart rate should normally be over sixty; below sixty, patients who were not trained athletes needed help. This patient's slow heart rate and low blood pressure were ominous signs of impending heart failure.

His heart needed a boost. Our standing orders dictated I start an IV and administer atropine to speed his heart rate.

If atropine didn't raise the heart rate, I was to inject epinephrine, a more aggressive drug, to kick up his heart's pumping.

Tanya had a non-rebreather mask on him with oxygen flowing at fifteen liters per minute. This provided 100% oxygen to the patient. I had the IV in his arm and had injected atropine when four firefighters stepped through the front door. His heart rate didn't change with the atropine, so I injected epinephrine.

"OK guys, we have a load-and-go, emergent, to the county ER. We need a driver. Please bring the gurney in ASAP."

"Got it, Sarge," a firefighter answered.

I jumped up and ran to the ambulance to prepare medications and the cardiac monitor. Firefighters and Tanya lifted the patient onto the gurney and hustled him to the ambulance.

They lined up the gurney with the rear of the ambulance and pushed. The wheels folded up and the gurney slid inside. As they lifted the gurney into the truck, the patient's left arm flopped off his chest. This, and his drooping eyelids, showed he was now only semi-conscious.

I said, "Hang in there, sir. We're going to get you to doctors right away. They are less than ten minutes from here."

His skin, now cool and clammy, were signs of shock. If we didn't stop this trend right away, he could slip into irreversible shock, where there was no coming back. He was still alive and breathing one hundred percent oxygen, but he no longer responded to me.

My patient was spiraling toward death.

I called out, "OK, driver, let's go, emergent, to county ER."

The driver lit up the emergency lights and whooped the siren through its four variations. He blasted the air horn every few seconds to clear traffic out of our way.

Tanya sat in the captain's chair as the driver started for the ER. She faced rearward at the patient's head, bagging him while assisting me by getting drugs and IV tubing between the breaths she pushed into him. I attached three cardiac monitor sticky-leads to his chest and saw a jagged sawtooth of a cardiac arrhythmia.

"Tanya, he's going into cardiac failure. I've got to tube him." *Tube him* meant pushing a tube down his throat and into his trachea and then bagging oxygen directly into his lungs.

Tanya climbed around me, trading places, and pulled out the intubation kit. In the cramped quarters of an ambulance, switching places resembled trying to walk in a row of seated theater spectators while the building shook in an earthquake.

Intubation is a delicate procedure. Too many patients died because an EMT mistakenly placed the tube in the larger, easier to reach esophagus. This pumped oxygen into the stomach, not the lungs. In a quiet operating room, an anesthesiologist and specialized nurse-anesthetist did this on a still table. I was doing it while careening down the road in an ambulance.

Holding the metal handle in my left hand, I pushed the curved blade with the tiny light on its tip to the back of his throat, lifting his lower jaw and tongue for a clear view. I looked for the V-shaped white vocal cords marking the entrance to his trachea. It took two tries. The diameter of an adult's trachea is usually smaller than the size of a pinky finger. I passed the airway tube through his cords, dropped the handle, attached a syringe to the tube, and inflated a balloon on the tip of the tube now near the patient's lungs—not allowing the tube to move even a millimeter. Tanya used her stethoscope over his stomach, then both sides of his chest, listening for sounds of air as I squeezed the Ambu-bag.

She confirmed, "No epigastric sounds and clear sounds left and right." She couldn't hear air entering his stomach. Clear sounds left and right meant the tube was placed perfectly.

Tanya secured the tube in place with tape. Jostling the patient might pull the tube out past the vocal cords or push it down into his left lung. We couldn't let it move as much as a quarter-inch.

"Take over bagging Tanya, good job..."

An insistent squealing alarm on the heart monitor drowned out my last word. Cardiac arrest!

"Shit! Tanya, we're losing him! Grab epinephrine syringes. Monitor times for me."

We climbed over each other so she could sit at his head and bag while getting supplies for me.

I had to compress the patient's chest about two times every second, then pause after thirty compressions while Tanya squeezed the Ambu-bag twice over six seconds. In those six seconds, I grabbed and opened a sealed package with a pre-filled epinephrine syringe, attached it to the IV port, pushed the drug in, then resumed compressions. We repeated epinephrine every three minutes.

"Tanya, please hand me the radio mic."

Years ago I read General Omar Bradley never issued an order without first saying please. I tried to imitate the General's habit; remembering to say it helped me remain calm. I didn't always remember. The unit's radio was on the wall behind Tanya, and she could reach it where I could not.

She handed the mic to me without interrupting her actions or her count of minutes and epinephrine doses.

I kept compressions going with a stiff left arm, using my weight to ensure adequate depth. Standing and doing proper stiff-armed compressions meant my head and shoulders were going up and down at least a third of the way through his chest. I looked like an oil field pump called a nodding donkey, but I pumped up and down a hundred times faster.

Keying the mic with my right hand, I said, "County ER, Unit-Five, emergency traffic, cardiac arrest."

Within a fraction of a second, a nurse's voice came back, "Unit Five, ER, go ahead with your transmission."

"ER, Unit-Five, inbound with severe, unstable respiratory distress, now in asystole with CPR in progress. I administered atropine and epinephrine on-scene. The patient is intubated, a thirty-two-year-old male. On-scene he was alert, diaphoretic, hypotensive, and bradycardic. The patient just crashed. ETA, standby ER..."

"Driver, what's our ETA?"

"Two minutes."

"ER, Unit Five continuing, ETA two minutes."

"Unit Five, ER, copy. ETA two minutes. Proceed immediately to room twelve. Over."

The driver gave us an outstanding arrival, stopping smoothly in the ambulance bay, causing Tanya and me only a slight stagger. A nurse ran outside to help as the firefighter opened the back door. The firefighter, Tanya, and nurse pulled the gurney out and to the ground. Clambering beside the gurney, I continued compressions, trying not to trip and fall from the truck.

I pumped his heart as best I could as his was no longer doing it for him.

We pushed into room twelve and slid the patient onto the ER bed. One nurse took over compressions, another confirmed good breath sounds after the move. I gave my full oral report to the doctor. Then Tanya, the firefighter, and I moved back to the doorway.

We watched the physician and nurses in the ER work hard to restart his heart, only to hear the doctor's words, "Time of death..."

What not to do after a gym workout? Die!

He was the second patient I lost in nine years as a paramedic. I walked out to the ambulance to restock supplies. I needed to be alone, needed to distract my mind from losing again. Tanya understood and left me to it.

Crew chiefs usually started paperwork, leaving restocking chores to partners. I went through the motions: checked the main oxygen tank; replaced the dirty airway equipment; got new IV bags, tubes, and needles from supply cabinets. Using a half quart of diluted bleach on the stretcher, I wiped it into the gurney pad's corners and underneath the rails. I threw a clean disposable sheet on the pad, making hospital corners and tucking them in. I smiled. Nurses laughed at me and my sheets. Hospital corners on sheets disappeared when nurses stopped wearing little white triangle hats and some genius invented fitted sheets.

After a half-hour, I wandered back into the ER. We had turned our patient over to our med-control doctor, an expert physician. He walked over to me saying, "I've been on the phone all this time to his brother, a cardiologist in New York. We've consulted on the data, and here's the truth, your patient was a dead-man-walking. His left anterior descending artery (known in medical circles as "the widow maker") was over ninety-five percent blocked. There was nothing you could have done to save him. Nothing you did hurt either."

"Nothing you did hurt." He said this knowing I blamed myself. He knew the standing orders I had followed—he had written them. The patient's heart was beating too slowly, too weakly, barely keeping him alive. I pushed drugs to strengthen and speed up his heart.

But, his body had tried to save itself from a failing heart by slowing the heart rate, reducing its workload. What his heart needed was a park bench; I gave drugs putting it in a one hundred yard dash.

I killed my second patient.

Yes, I did what the standing orders—our protocols—said I should do. The following year the orders were revised by the doctor. In this newer version we had to do a more sophisticated twelve-lead EKG before giving drugs in patients with severe respiratory distress or slow heart rates. A twelve-lead EKG showed if an acute cardiac condition caused the distress. If so, speeding the heart could be fatal. The doctor recognized we make mistakes. We learn from them. We change what we do. Then move on. He was better at moving on than I.

I had lived sixty years with the belief I would never lose to Death because I would do things right. I would beat Death and make up for not saving my sister. A few months ago, Santa shook my belief. Now, the foundation for my career choices began crumbling. Could I really beat Death?

His mocking presence sent a chill up my spine. Did I hear him say, *"There will be more calls. We'll meet again,"* or did I imagine it?

2015- A Routine Checkup

Exhausted, my partner Bobby and I staggered into the musty concrete-block EMS substation Five. We had run six back-to-back calls, leaving us limp as wet dishcloths, low-bloodsugar-hungry, behind on paperwork. We were only a third of the way through our twelve-hour shift.

I thought again of how much I needed this day to be peaceful, of how I had walked into the substation at first light with hands clasped together in the act of praying for a quiet shift, and of how, for all that, we had been dispatched immediately, without coffee, to a cardiac arrest.

Bobby drawled, "Sarge, all I want is a few minutes of quiet to catch my breath. Then I'll go wash the truck and complete our checkoff. You take it easy, OK?"

Bobby never failed to wash an ambulance with soap and water every shift he worked.

"Bobby, you are part duck and enjoy getting wet. I'll finish my checkoff inside the truck while you wash the outside."

A 911 ambulance carries perhaps a thousand, maybe more, individual items, ranging from a band-aid to the jaws of life. Policy dictated a crew touch, count, check every single item at the start of every shift. Two shifts per day. And the truck was to be washed each shift.

"Unit Seven, County, emergency traffic!"

Our radios interrupted the quiet like a breaking glass. We both startled and turned the volume down on our radios. We carried the speaker-mics clipped to our shirts near our ears. There had been no alert tone, so we knew right away the call was for a different unit. The alert tone sounded like a weather warning. This time, they called Unit Seven—we were Unit Five.

I said, "Forget the truck washing partner, we'll be heading to standby inside five minutes."

Bobby asked, "Are Units Seven and Ten paramedic crews?" Those two units were the only two covering the county's northern region.

"I don't know. County will send somebody to fill in for them, and we're the closest paramedic crew. So I expect it will be us."

Bobby drawled his response in his best John Wayne imitation, "Yeah, Sarge. They cain't let us catch a breath, can they?"

Bobby is deep-south, lean and fit, in his early forties. His friends described Bobby as practical, accustomed to hard work, ready to move when needed. Whether walking or driving, he normally started moving slow and careful, accelerated to the speed limit, then when needed continued until reaching NASCAR speed. Every paramedic in our Service looked forward to a shift with him. We couldn't ask for a better wingman.

We sat in the station recliners and listened with ears glued to our radios like blue jays on the ground in a backyard listen for an approaching cat—alert, nervous, never completely relaxing.

"County, Unit Seven is responding."

"Unit Seven, truck versus auto, I-26 westbound, mile marker 93, eight vehicles, overturn."

I-26—the major east-west interstate to and from the state capital.

Without a pause, Dispatch called out the shift supervisor, "Supervisor, County, emergency traffic, I-26 westbound."

Calling out the captain-supervisor meant a multi-casualty, multi-jurisdictional incident involving fire, police, and EMS. Thankfully, this only happened maybe once in twelve months.

Before the supervisor could respond on the radio, Dispatch sent another call-out, "Unit Ten, County, emergency traffic, I-26 westbound." Dispatching Unit Ten, the other ambulance covering the north, stripped that area of EMS coverage.

"Damn Bobby! I-26 will be a parking lot what with weekend rush hour traffic heading home. We need to head that way. We'll be on standby or the interstate ourselves."

"Unit Five, Supervisor. Standby in the Bi-Lo lot." The Bi-Lo grocery store shared a parking lot with a Burger King.

"OK, Sarge. We caught a break—standby instead of going to the interstate. We can grab a drink and a burger. I'm starved. Been wanting to eat since the shift started. What do you think?"

"I think the minute food hits our mouths dispatch will call us. Let's keep our fingers crossed." Neither of us had brought lunches with us this day.

Bobby drove us north to our standby point while I rested my head against the passenger door window. We were a mile from the parking lot, a mile from a cold drink and food, when it came.

"Unit Five, County, emergency traffic."

Bobby answered, "County, Unit Five responding."

"Unit Five, County, patient transport from doctor's office."

The address on the computer screen showed the doctor's office next door to a community-based Urgent Care and Surgery Center. When patients walked into the doctor's office and not the Urgent Care, that almost always meant they weren't critical. As tired as we were, we welcomed this transport as nothing more than a high-tech taxi ride to a hospital.

Doctors occasionally called for an ambulance to transport a patient to a hospital for further tests, or sometimes to be admitted overnight. Private ambulance services were supposed to handle these calls, but often needed an hour before being available. Doctors knew a call to 911 would have an ambulance there in minutes.

"Bobby, pull up to the back door. God forbid patients in the front lobby see an ambulance crew taking a patient out of a doctor's office for medical care."

"Sure thing, Sarge."

Pulling into the parking lot, Bobby said, "Look Sarge, two nurses are holding the door open. This looks like an easy one. We don't even need the jump bag."

The jump bag— a 75 pound, 3-foot long duffle crammed with emergency equipment, ranging from bandaids to oxygen masks to cardiac drugs. Bringing it made pushing and maneuvering a patient-loaded stretcher twice as difficult.

"All right, Bobby, we'll leave the jump bag."

Nurses rarely met us with an open door. Ordinarily, we would bang on the heavy metal door loud enough for someone to hear us in the labyrinth of hallways and exam rooms. Two nurses were unheard of; I guessed they were taking a break, maybe a smoke break.

Bobby parked the ambulance next to the nurses. We got out and opened the rear ambulance doors and took out our rolling gurney. Bobby lifted the jump bag from it and dumped it on the bench seat in the patient compartment. We followed the nurses into the building. They weren't talking or hurrying, just nonchalantly passing closed exam rooms lining the hallway.

As we walked a half-dozen steps down the empty hallway, it hit me: *where's the staff?* Just a fleeting shadow of wondering, almost a sensation, had me thinking, *this is odd.* And I dismissed it.

Ooomph, Ooomph, Ooomph. Those sounds came from ahead of us. Bobby turned to me, frowning, lips pressed into a thin line. I frowned, mirroring his look. *That sounds like CPR. But that makes no sense. Dispatch sent us for a simple transport, not a cardiac arrest. There are no shouts, no orders, no urgent voices. These nurses aren't hurrying. They didn't mention a problem, let alone an arrest.* We continued on, puzzled, now uneasy. The hair on the back of my neck prickled as a sense of foreboding squeezed my gut.

We turned into the last room, and the scene slammed me in the face. It is CPR! Oh Lord, this can't be real! And we're standing here naked without our equipment! *Shit! Shit! Shit!*

Four or five nurses stood in a semicircle around a doctor in her white lab coat, all intent upon another nurse straddling a wisp of a woman on an exam table—the nurse doing chest compressions, making an Ooomph, Ooomph, Ooomph sound as air pushed from the patient. The woman on the receiving end of the compressions had a sun-weathered face, looking to be anywhere from forty to her mid-fifties. Strands of dark hair interrupting gray bounced with each compression on her chest.

Bobby stopped frozen in mid-stride, eyes widening.

When the unexpected lands on you, you don't waste time questioning, wondering how or why. That can come later. What you do is assess the situation, evaluate the downsides and upsides, decide what needs to be done, figure out how, and do it.

"Bobby, get the jump bag and monitor from the unit!"

I needed the cardiac monitor with its built-in EKG and defibrillator. He disappeared in an instant, his boots squeaking on the polished hall floor as he sprinted back down the hallway to get the equipment.

Keying my radio, I called, "County, Unit Five. Cardiac Arrest! Send backup, emergent! Send a driver too."

We needed a firefighter to drive us to the hospital so Bobby could help me with the patient in the back of the truck.

"Unit Five, County. Be advised, all fire units are at the interstate scene, and no other county units are available."

No backup! Not even the supervisor who is at the interstate.

That nurse is doing compressions without an oxygen mask on the patient! She's not even doing mouth-to-mouth!

I tapped the nurse doing CPR on the shoulder, moving her off the table as I took over chest compressions, pumping hard and fast. I stood over six feet tall and didn't need to climb up on the exam table like the nurse had done.

The doctor outranked me by miles, but stood quietly and out of the way. She apparently was overjoyed to let me take over and assume responsibility. Doctors letting us take over was common when an emergency happened outside a hospital. They could only keep control of patient care by maintaining personal responsibility and riding with us in the ambulance to the ER.

I shot multiple questions toward the doctor, "How long have you been doing CPR? Don't you have any oxygen?"

The doctor replied, "We've been at this about fifteen minutes. We don't keep oxygen masks here in the office."

A five-dollar rescue oxygen mask! What the hell is wrong with a medical practice that doesn't have a basic oxygen mask? Unbelievable! The situation was crashing around me, and I took pride in keeping my thoughts to myself.

Bobby burst into the room carrying a hundred pounds of monitor-plus-jump-bag.

I said, "Partner, get the BVM, insert an airway, and start bagging! Hook up to our O2."

We equipped every gurney with a portable twenty-minute oxygen tank.

The standard method for providing rescue breathing to a patient was with a BVM, bag-valve-mask. When I paused chest compressions after thirty, Bobby inserted the J-shaped plastic airway device into her mouth and throat to keep the tongue from closing her airway. With his left hand he clamped a form-fitting mask over the patient's mouth and nose and with his other hand squeezed the bag twice to breathe for her.

"Bobby, the next time you bag, I'll step around you, attach the monitor to her, and get an EKG."

The doctor and nurses remained back, watching silently.

In the six seconds he took to push two breaths, I grabbed a package of chest leads from a side pocket on the monitor, ripped open the foil package, ripped open the patient's blouse, attached the EKG leads to her chest, and plugged the leads into our heart monitor. Immediately, the screen showed the ominous flat line! *Shocks wouldn't work!* I resumed compressions.

We got into our rhythm—thirty compressions, pause for two BVM breaths, three seconds each, then start another thirty compressions.

Grunting as I worked I said, "Bobby, I don't know how we are getting this lady to the ER by ourselves. Do you have any ideas?"

"How about these nurses help slide her onto our stretcher, then I drive while you do CPR? Who knows how long it will be before there is backup available."

This can't end well! If I do one-person CPR while Bobby drives, I can't start an IV, give drugs, or do anything else to pull her back. Not good!

A three-person ambulance crew appeared in the doorway! Vito, the paramedic on Unit Ten, Tanya, and a firefighter. Vito said, "We heard your call for backup, and I knew there were no fire units available. The supervisor cleared us from the accident on I-26. What do you want us to do? I've got a firefighter ride-along with us today."

A miracle! Not only did a top-notch crew show up, but they also brought the rare firefighter spending the day with them for a ride-along.

"Take over CPR while I start an IV and push epi. Your firefighter can be our driver."

Epi—epinephrine—the standard heart stimulating drug we would give every three minutes. It's the same chemical the body uses to cause heartbeats.

Vito started compressions, Tanya opened jump bag compartments for me, lining up supplies and drugs, Bobby kept on bagging.

Within ninety seconds, I had done what usually took four minutes: grabbed the supplies, started an IV in a vein, drew up the epinephrine into a syringe, then injected it into the IV.

The flat line remained unchanged on the EKG monitor.

As the paramedic in charge, I called out orders, "Help us get her onto the stretcher and out to our unit. She can't weigh but eighty or ninety pounds. At the next pause, we move her. On three, ready? One, two, three," and we lifted her from the exam table to the stretcher without missing more than a single compression.

"OK, let's head out! Driver, please open the door for us, then get into the front and radio to Dispatch." Tanya and I pushed the stretcher while Vito continued compressions and Bobby kept up bagging with oxygen attached.

We rushed the gurney out to the truck. I climbed up into the unit to take over compressions. Vito and Tanya pushed the gurney in as Bobby climbed up and settled into the rear-facing Captain's chair to continue airway management and bagging.

Vito and Tanya climbed in and Vito took over compressions as I managed the cardiac monitor. The truck swayed and the driver's door slammed as the firefighter climbed into the driver's seat.

The driver said, "County, Unit Five is en route to County ER, emergent, with a cardiac arrest. Firefighter-driver is on board."

"Bobby, you maintain steady bagging. Tanya, can you set up a saline drip for me? Thanks."

Suddenly, the EKG changed to a fast heartbeat. Vito and I stared, speechless for a second. Flat lines rarely changed to normal-looking rhythms, maybe once in fifty arrests.

"Look Vito! We're showing a sinus tachycardia. Check for a pulse!"

The heart sends electrical signals to its muscles and we see those electrical pulses on the EKG, but heart muscles may not respond with an effective heartbeat. We call this a P-E-A—pulseless electrical activity. Even though the EKG shows electrical impulses going to the heart's chambers, the heart isn't beating, and the patient is still dead. We had to feel a pulse every time the monitor showed a spike. A sinus tachycardia looked like a fast but normal heartbeat, something healthy joggers or cyclists experience when going all out.

Vito leaned over the patient and placed two fingers on the side of her neck, feeling for a carotid pulse. "We've got it! Rapid, weak, but definite. We got her back! We've got ROSC."

ROSC—Return Of Spontaneous Circulation. The patient's heart beating on its own, the best possible news following a cardiac arrest.

"OK," I said, "We have a pulse! Let's go. Thanks a load, guys, you saved our bacon."

Her heart beat on its own, circulating the oxygen Bobby pushed into her.

Vito and Tanya needed to be released to cover their region. They climbed out, and our driver took off for the ER. Bobby had to keep bagging with the BVM; the patient had a good heartbeat but wasn't breathing on her own. Apprehensive, watching for any change signaling an impending crash, I stayed edgy, eyes glued to the heart monitor.

I grabbed the radio handset mounted on the cabin wall and transmitted, "County ER, Unit Five is inbound, emergent, with a cardiac arrest. We've achieved ROSC after a total of thirty-five minutes of CPR, IV established, one epi, and sinus tachycardia at 127. ETA eleven minutes."

"Unit Five, County ER, copy and standing by."

"We did it, Sarge!"

Feeling as euphoric as teammates in a dressing room after winning the championship game, Bobby and I high-fived. We had done what we signed up for! We marveled at the simple fact we saved her. A few minutes ago, she was dead, and now she lived. We had done it right.

Almost right. When we got back to our station, the after-action review began. "You know we screwed up, right Bobby?"

"Yep. There's a reason it's policy to always carry the jump bag into the scene. We barely missed a disaster."

"Bobby, let me tell you a story. My Grandfather Carl, an engineer from pure German stock, could fix anything. My dad called him a genius with hand-tools. I was seven the last time I visited him. One day, Grandpa Carl let me help him fix a dripping outdoor faucet.

He picked up his toolbox. It must have weighed over seventy-five pounds, like our jump bag. When we got to the faucet, he used three tools: a Philips screwdriver, pliers, and an open-end wrench. When we got back to his workbench, I asked him why he carried the whole toolbox out when he only used three tools.

Grandpa Carl said, 'Dave, I didn't know what else I might have to do once I got there, did I? It's best to have your tools with you. If you don't, you are likely to find something you didn't expect, and you'll get frustrated and discouraged.'

It's too bad I didn't remember his wise advice."

The following day the captain stepped into our station. He didn't meet our eyes. He sat down, staring at his hands in his lap.

"The family took your patient off life-support this morning. She had gone too long without oxygen; she was brain-dead. You should feel grateful you gave the family time to say their goodbyes."

After four minutes of not breathing, brain cells are dying. After six minutes, the brain dies en masse, the lights go out, the door closes forever.

Should I be grateful I gave the family time to say goodbye? I saw it as me dumping the burden on them of deciding to pull the plug and saying out loud to another human being, "Unplug the machines and let her die."

Something ripped out of me. What's the point of all the training and study and work if we couldn't give this woman a life worth living? Something big changed. I needed to define it, put words to it, but it floated away like a soap bubble until it popped and disappeared. I tried to remember what it was, but it seemed to slide just out of my reach of remembering.

I must catch whatever changed, or I too will fade away.

I couldn't save them all.

With every critical patient I would tell myself, *but I'll save this one.* And when I saved them, it was everything I needed. Except here, Death ripped it away in the most painful way possible, leaving only a husk of a body.

I finally realized the something breaking that day, floating away—was the reason I became a paramedic, the belief I could beat Death.

Trying to beat Death is folly. Thinking I can is nothing more than a sorry-assed fairy-tale. Trying to erase the past is fighting an unwinnable battle. All the while I thought I was winning, Death watched and waited, mocking me. It's his sick joke to let me think I'm winning when I am really losing.

I understood all at once I wasn't beating anything, certainly not Death. If I won, it was because Death let me. And no matter how many lives I might save, they would not, could not, erase my slate. I had been holding onto the nine-year-old's belief. Now I saw this belief as a lie, but what was the truth?

In the two years spent on the street after the woman in the doctor's office, I never again wanted to know a patient's outcome. It was just better to focus on my job of getting them to the ER alive.

2016- The Last Call

5:00 P.M., EST (1700 hours)

Friday, five o'clock in the afternoon. Businesses and offices are closing. Workers clear their desks, powering off desktop computers. Ceremonies come to an end. Drivers are getting into their cars and starting the race for home.

Tanya was my partner on this day, my last day as a paramedic working for the County. The end of yet another career. We were relaxing in the EMS ready room, having spent the day without a single call. We sat side-by-side in recliners and reminisced about the years and calls we had shared.

"Papa, if you could change some policy, what would it be?"

"I would change our policy of rotating partners, and I would assign you and Bobby as my permanent wingmen. Sorry, wingpersons."

"Why would you do that?"

"If you remember, I was guarding nuclear fuel when I joined the service. Experience taught me to pair security officers as permanent partners, like modern police departments do. My most trusted sergeants, Ray and his wife Patti, were my A-team. Ray was a retired detective who had survived more than his share of gunfights. Patti was a deliciously fiery red-head. They knew each other's moves so well they appeared to be dancing through trouble. They could communicate with each other by a glance, by the merest movement of a hand. When the situation goes sideways and there isn't time for a discussion, permanent partners survive longer than temporaries."

Tanya said, "Well, you know why the chief wants to rotate partners. That solves two problems for him. First, it minimizes personnel conflicts when two EMTs can't play nice together. Second, it minimizes personnel issues when two EMTs play too nicely together in station bedrooms. We've seen more than three broken marriages and a half-dozen EMT's fired for screwing around."

"Yeah, that's one way to solve two problems, rather than making partners get along and behave."

We lapsed into silence for several minutes. Could I be so lucky to end a decade plus career as a street medic without breaking a sweat? This day wasn't as exciting as most, but at this stage of my career I was very much into boring routine. I had enough excitement to last several lifetimes.

Tanya said, "What are you thinking about now?"

"You mean besides a quiet shift? Do you remember that woman who died in the doctor's office, the call where you and Vito backed me up? We celebrated getting her heart beating once again. Later we learned the doctor's staff left her brain dead, doing fifteen minutes of CPR without giving her oxygen.

"Since then, I did a lot of questioning of my purpose. Like most of us, I devoted myself to saving lives, to beating Death. This is my thing, Tanya, this is what I'm built for. I'm a medic, always was, always will be. I'm a hunter of disease and trauma.

But that call made me realize saving a life isn't always the best thing, or maybe not even the right thing to do."

With half-open eyes, Tanya said, "Papa, that's way too heavy for your last shift. One-hundred-twenty minutes until you're retired. Two hours and you won't have to jump up for another 911 call. What are your plans?"

"Plans? I always said my wake would be my retirement party. I never planned to retire from being a paramedic. As the saying goes, I thought I would die with my boots on. Now it's just two hours until I'm forced to. Forced to take over for my wife in her last few months of raising our granddaughter. Of running our house. Of living."

Tanya and Bobby were the only two partners who knew about my wife Ellie's battle with cancer. I didn't share that with others. It was a losing battle, and I would soon take compassionate leave, followed by retirement.

Tanya said, "I'm so sorry you have to go through this. How long have you two been married?"

"Twenty-five years. We met and became friends, business friends, as my first marriage of thirty years disintegrated. It was only after being friends for two years and after my divorce that we started our romance. She's given me one helluva great ride.

"Honestly, Tanya, I don't know how I'll do it. I can't picture myself not working. Hell, that's what I've done since graduating high school over a half century ago. But it is what it is. I have to stay home and take over for Ellie. She isn't strong enough to lift the kid anymore. You know, Aubri turned eleven this year, and picking her up and down out of her wheelchair, the toilet, the bed, is getting too much for Ellie."

Tanya reached over and touched my arm. She said, "Ellie is an awesome lady. I'm sorry."

"Yes, she is."

We fell silent after that and closed our eyes. But we wouldn't fall asleep, as sleep wasn't allowed during twelve-hour shifts.

5:15 P.M., EST (1715 hours)

Rush hour traffic is getting more congested, less patient, more frustrated. Tired workers-now-drivers are getting crankier.

The setting sun slides down inch by inch on westbound windshields, approaching the bottom edges of visors lowered to shade drivers' eyes as they head for home.

"You know Tanya, you've been a terrific partner, and we've worked a lot of calls together, tough calls, easy calls, quickies and a few that went on for hours. But you've been an even better friend. I'll miss you, miss washing these trucks, running calls, hearing about your family."

"You liar! You will not miss washing these trucks."

"I suppose you're right. Listen girl, I don't want you to tell anyone else about this. Nobody knows but the captains and the chief. I've been diagnosed with cancer myself. I'll start radiation and chemo in a few months, and I've been warned that will sap too much energy for me to continue working on the street."

"Aw shit, Papa! I'm so sorry. I'll be over whenever you need me."

She meant it, even believed it. We had worked together for what, ten years? But at her age Tanya could have been my daughter, even a granddaughter. I appreciated her intention, but I knew we would lose touch as we swirled in our separate courses through this whirlpool of life.

My wife attracted friends like a magnet attracted iron filings. She was a friend magnet. Even so, only two remained in touch with her from her school days. I didn't have any who stayed in touch with me. My EMS buddies jokingly called me a shit magnet.

And that was okay. Aubri needed twenty-four-seven care because of her Cerebral Palsy. I wouldn't have time for friends.

5:30 P.M., EST (1730 hours)

On Harmon Road, the eighteen-wheel-semi driver heads east toward downtown and his depot. Harmon Road is two lanes wide. Vehicle side mirrors traveling opposite directions miss by a foot or two. The trucker is making good time, maybe edging just over the legal limit of forty-five mph. Downtown is still forty minutes away for him. He was tired, and hungry, and thirsty, and in need of the bathroom, and behind schedule. And frustrated.

Once he got back to his depot, he had another twenty minutes of cleaning his truck and paperwork before clocking out. Drivers had to complete paperwork during regular shift time, otherwise it was on their own time.

The sun drops, inch by inch, stretching shadows longer and longer.

The woman driving west on Harmon Road is no longer shaded as the sun flares beneath the edge of her visor.

Her world implodes as 38,000 pounds of semi pulverizes her 5,600 pounds of SUV. Shrapnel of auto glass sprays outward and inward from every window of her vehicle. There are no squeals of locked tires on the road, not from the semi, not from her SUV, as they meet head-on.

Sixty G's crush her body down and under the dashboard, around the brake and accelerator pedals. The SUV's rear end continues westward at 60 mph, crushing everything behind the driver's seat like it was cardboard instead of steel. The front seats continue forward until they crunch into the dashboard.

Her crash is over in seventy milliseconds, except for the falling dust and dying echoes. Seventy milliseconds? Cut a second in half, that is five hundred milliseconds. Split that in half again, two-hundred-fifty milliseconds. Cut in half again, one-hundred-twenty-five. Take half once more, and her crash is over. One-half of one-half of one-half of one-half of a second.

Still 5:30 P.M., EST (1730 hours)

"A quiet shift, not too bad for your last one, eh Papa?"

"Darn it Tanya. You know better than to brag about a quiet shift. You'll jinx us for sure if the EMS Goddess hears you."

She laughed.

I said, "But, no, not bad at all. I guess that's why the captain put me down here on Unit Three. He thought my last shift should be a quiet one, after all the crazy calls. Do you think they'll miss me, or will they even notice I'm gone?"

"Come on, Papa, you know dang well they'll miss you. Especially your smart-aleck radio traffic, like the time you told dispatch our GPS was FUBAR. We could hear crews laughing all over the county. They couldn't believe you said it on the radio. By the way, did the captain say anything to you about saying FUBAR?"

"Yes, he called me at home after the shift. He asked if I knew what FUBAR meant. I said yes, fouled up beyond all repair. Naturally, I cleaned it up and tried really hard not to let him hear me laugh..."

The alarm tone sounded on our radios and a second later Dispatch broadcast, "Unit Three, County, emergency traffic."

"Tanya, I said you would jinx us! I'll drive. This should be my last call, and I get to play with the lights and siren." Then, keying my radio mic clipped to my shoulder epaulet , "County, Unit Three is en route."

"Unit Three, County. Head-on auto versus truck, Harmon Road."

All serious now, I said, "County, Unit Three is responding emergent to a head-on collision, Harmon Road."

Tanya and I stood and headed out of the station to our unit.

We climbed into the ambulance and started toward the crash. Emergency lights strobed bright and the siren wailed. I drove for the last time.

"OK, Tanya, be sure to put on your traffic vest. If we're first on the scene, I'll take incident command, you'll be in charge of patient care. If Fire is there already, they'll have command. In that case you and I will separate and triage if there are several vehicles involved."

Tanya was a consummate professional, and I didn't need to tell her what to do. I only talked out loud to be sure we were both on the same page, a technique learned years earlier.

"You got it, Papa. Shoot! Look—westbound traffic's backed up turning onto Harmon. They aren't moving at all. The left shoulder is clear though; it looks like no oncoming traffic is getting through up ahead."

We turned left onto Harmon and I drove west on the wrong side of the road—the side empty of traffic.

I said, " I can see fire engines blocking traffic up there. Look Tanya. Damn, that truck is an eighteen-wheeler! It doesn't look damaged though. Maybe this won't be too bad."

Seconds later Tanya exclaimed, "Shit, look at that wreck on the right shoulder. I can't even tell what kind of car it was. I guess this is bad after all."

Pulling as close as I could behind fire engines, I radioed, "County, Unit Three is on scene reporting to Command. Place the helicopter on standby, please."

I snatched the small trauma bag and jumped down to the street. Tanya got out and rushed to the rear ambulance compartment to bring the bigger seventy-five pound jump bag.

I hustled over to the destroyed car, my boots crunching on the windshield's fragments carpeting the roadway, and I sidestepped a rainbow puddle of gasoline and radiator fluid. The low sun was full on my face forcing me to squint at the carnage.

Firefighters scrambled, using pry bars, trying in vain to get to occupants.

The car's roof crushed down through the windshield, down to the door handles. There were no side windows left, only crumpled sheet metal. The space where the windshield used to be was now a hole only twelve inches high. The car doors would never open again. The car's rear end had accordioned through the back passenger area and pushed into the backs of the front seats.

More firefighters carried the jaws-of-life to cut open the crumpled roof.

The Fire Chief, acting as incident commander, pointed through the windshield space, and said, "The driver is a woman. You can just see her head under the steering wheel. We can't get to her."

Stepping onto the top of a front-wheel tire that leaned out at a forty-five degree angle, I crawled onto the crumpled hood, pushing glass pebbles out of my way, cutting my knees on those I missed, and made my way to where the windshield should have been. My job was to keep driver and passengers alive and protected while firefighters worked to free them.

I looked down through the steering wheel to see a small, pale face turned toward the passenger seat. Her left eye, the one I could see, was closed, her head pinned to the seat by the the steering wheel. The rest of her was hidden under the dashboard, crushed into a space no bigger than a briefcase. I pulled off my Kevlar hazmat glove and slid my arm through the steering wheel to check for a carotid pulse. There was no pulse, no breathing. I believed she died within milliseconds after her car met the truck's front bumper.

"County, Unit Three, signal nine at seventeen forty-hours. Cancel the chopper." I realized that if there had been anyone in the rear seat, they would also be dead.

Signal nine—I pronounced her dead, using the County's coded phrase to avoid the word "dead" on open airwaves. I silently thanked God I didn't see any blood; the dash hid the hideous trauma. What I could see looked serene; she could have been asleep. I strained to block imagined images of her body.

I climbed down from the car's hood as the Fire Chief stepped close. I forced a controlled tone into my voice.

"Any other passengers?"

"Not that we've seen, Sergeant. There are no side or back windows left for us to look through. Once we peel back the roof, we'll confirm."

When was the last time anyone called me Sergeant? I realized then I didn't recognize him; he was new in this area. And he didn't know me yet, hence the formality.

She had been driving west, possibly on her way home from work after five o'clock. She had the sun in her eyes, but could she miss a whale-sized truck? Had she been texting?

I crossed to the opposite roadside where the truck driver stood in front of his rig, talking with a County deputy.

The driver turned to me and said, "I'm not hurt, I'm okay."

He turned back to the deputy and said, "I was driving the speed limit, you know, forty-five, and she just veered into my lane. I couldn't stop. There wasn't enough time to avoid her."

Tanya looked into the car as she approached us. She winced and turned away.

I said, "Tanya, the truck driver is okay; he's not injured. We don't know if there is anyone else in the car. Even if there is, we won't need the jump bag equipment. There won't be any survivors. Just copy down what information you can about the woman's identity. Cops will give you whatever they learn when they run a make on her license plate or VIN number, when they find it."

"Sure, Sarge." What she had seen turned her into a woman of few words.

"Hey Sarge," a firefighter who knew me called. "Look at this."

They had pried open a three-foot hole in the car's roof over the back seat, curling the metal back like opening a can of sardines. As I walked over, the firefighter lifted a United States flag from the back seat. The flag was folded into a precise triangle. No red showing. I immediately thought, *a military funeral fold.*

"There's no one else in the car, Sarge. Just this folded flag sitting on the seat. The impact pushed the back seat right against the front seat, and the flag couldn't go anywhere."

I thought, *she was returning from a funeral. Maybe she was crying, with tears blurring her vision. The VA and its cemetery were east of here, and she was driving west.* Suddenly, I imagined her aiming for the front of that eighteen-wheeler. Nobody drives with a burial flag on the back seat. Not even for a few days.

The deputy found the license plate, and got her basic information from her DMV record. He said to me, "She was born in 1966."

That made her fifty years old, give or take some months. The flag could be for her husband, a son or daughter. I would never find out.

As I stared at the flag, the scene faded from the accident to an imagined funeral.

I watch as an Honor Guard lifts the burial flag draping the casket of a deceased veteran. They place the flag on a closed casket with the union blue field over the deceased's left shoulder. I hear Taps, and the Honor Guard folds the flag into a symbolic tri-cornered shape. A properly folded flag will fold thirteen times on the triangles. This represents the thirteen original colonies. The folded flag symbolizes a tri-cornered hat worn by the

*American Revolution Patriots. Once folded correctly, no red or white stripe
is showing, leaving only the blue field with stars.*

*With these words the honor guard presents the flag to her as next
of kin: "On behalf of the President of the United States, and a grateful
Nation, please accept this flag as a symbol of our appreciation for your
loved one's honorable and faithful service."*

"Papa, are you all right?" Tanya's whisper brought me back to
Harmon Road. I stood in the middle of the street with the wind
flattening my pants against my legs.

I nodded and said, "I guess we're done here. Let's head back to the
station and finish the report."

6:50 P.M., EST (1850 hours)

Back at Station Three, Tanya and I sat quietly, spending the last
ten minutes of my career reflecting on calls we shared, avoiding talking
about this last call.

"What are you thinking about, Papa?"

"You know, Tanya, I spent my life thinking I had to save lives, I had
to beat Death, to atone for my sister. I was wrong. At nine years old,
running from the fire was the only sensible thing to do. We can't change
the past. We can't atone, no matter how many lives we save."

A tear glistened in Tanya's eye and she lowered her head to gaze at
her hands in her lap. She gently rubbed her hands over and over, as if
washing them.

"The two patients I lost, Santa and the gym patient? I didn't kill
them. They only died in my care because I followed flawed protocols.
Their deaths put a spotlight on the flaws, which were then fixed.

"The woman who died in the doctor's office? I learned saving a life
can be contrary to the natural order of things. That woman taught me
to see death, not an apparition that I named Death, who was my enemy.

"And this last woman? I think she found peace. I think she saw
death as a friend. Was it an accident? Did she accidentally hit a huge
semi head-on, and not some family van?"

6:55 P.M., EST (1855 hours)

Tanya and I sat quietly, contemplative, her hand holding mine. The clock on the station wall ticked to the end of my last shift.

"Papa, what will you be doing for the next few weeks?"

"I'm taking Ellie and Aubri on a week-long trip to Ellie's high school reunion in Mansfield, Ohio. Aubri will stay with us at Bubba's house, Ellie's lifelong classmate and closest friend. Afterward, perhaps I'll do part-time paralegal work from the house."

"Oh yeah, which reunion is it?"

"Her last."

At once, I regretted blurting it like that.

"Her fiftieth. Her class only holds reunions every five years now, and Ellie hasn't missed a single one. It's special for her, like going home—where she grew up with family and friends she cherished."

"I hope you have a good time."

2016- A Busman's Holiday

Ellie and I hadn't taken a vacation in over sixteen years, not since moving from California to South Carolina. We gave up our West Coast business, home, family, and friends to help care for her aging mother on the East Coast. The last trip we took was a decade ago, to escort Ellie's mother to her funeral, held in her home state of Ohio, her hometown of Mansfield—a trip, not a vacation.

A month after the funeral in 2005, we took on twenty-four-seven care of Ellie's great granddaughter Aubri, then four months old, born with brain damage and Cerebral Palsy. I worked days as a tactical commander of a security force guarding nuclear fuel rods, and took a second full-time job as an EMT, working nights, to replace Ellie's substitute teacher income, which she gave up to stay with the baby.

Ten years later Ellie's high school reunion beckoned. She was going to celebrate fifty years since her graduation. Ellie had attended every reunion, held once every five years. She let me know missing the big fifty wasn't an option.

Ellie tended toward the stoic, not given to displays of emotion. But in her excitement over this reunion, she hummed like electricity buzzing through power lines.

She announced, "I'm shopping today for new clothes. I'm getting you something nicer than the old suit you wore to Mom's funeral."

I said, "All right, a blazer or sport coat." Clothes shopping bored me to annoyance. But this wasn't a battle I chose to argue.

She came home several hours later, practically prancing with excitement. She presented her prize: two new dresses, one for the semi-formal dinner, and for me a new sport jacket, dress shirt, and slacks, making an ensemble. I had argued my fifteen-year-old ties were good enough. She picked the one tie out of two dozen she would allow me to wear in front of her high school friends.

We took a week's vacation and drove to Mansfield where she grew up. A group of Ellie's classmates planned the reunion down to the hour.

Wednesday would be school tours, meeting teachers in classrooms, and a cafeteria lunch. Thursday, graduates and guests could visit nearby towns and local memory venues such as the old ice cream parlor where students hung out after school. The planning committee left Friday afternoon free. Friday night featured the homecoming football game. Saturday night we would enjoy the reunion dinner—the closing event. The committee rented a community center, a four-piece band, and caterers for the dinner-dance.

The week lived up to Ellie's highest expectations, and she thrilled at renewing acquaintances and friendships. The capstone Saturday night dinner started with name tags as guests lined up at a reception table. Videos of their original graduation ceremony played on monitors suspended from the ceiling. A bar served drinks, a few couples danced to Oldies-but-Goodies. After the last of guests arrived, caterers served dinners at round tables-for-six. The servers arranged the tables in a horseshoe shape around a dance floor big enough for ten couples. The band played at a conversational volume from a riser the height of an apple box. A photographer walked the hall snapping portraits.

Forty-five minutes into dinner, a woman hurried to the bandstand. She motioned to the band to stop, took the microphone, and said, "Is there a doctor in the house?"

Damn. I held my breath, looked around the audience, but no one stood, raised a hand, or asked why. I thought I heard a pin drop.

Here I sat with no partner or equipment. I was off duty and outside my jurisdiction. This put me in a legal no-man's-land, trapped between being an ordinary citizen and a trained professional. Good Samaritan laws protect a citizen. But courts hold trained professionals to higher legal standards. If I volunteered, my dilemma became: risk being jailed for practicing medicine without a license, or risk being sued by a family for not doing enough.

I sat at the dinner table turning this over in my mind for a second-and-a-half. It felt like a blink of an eye, but was long enough for my wife to whisper, "Aren't you going to do something?"

Please let a doctor come forward, or at least another professional. This didn't happen.

My throat went dry, my face went hot. But with Ellie's words urging me on, I rose, crossed the dance floor to the woman on the bandstand and said, "I'm a paramedic. What's wrong?"

The woman said, "Follow me, a gentleman has collapsed out in the corridor."

We walked quickly toward double doors to the corridor, left the dining hall, and turned left. He lay, face up, his sport coat open, his tie falling across a shoulder. He wasn't wearing the white jacket of a server, so I took him to be another reunion guest. Kneeling, I checked his neck for a pulse as I bent my ear to his nose, looking down his torso for chest rise.

No pulse.

No breathing!

He was warm, pink, and dead.

I ripped his shirt open splashing buttons in all directions. Starting CPR immediately, his ribs popped and the half-dozen people gathered around gasped.

"Can someone please get me a cloth dinner napkin?" The watch-and-wait days after years ago doing unprotected mouth-to-mouth on a baby—worried I had caught HIV or meningitis—taught me a hard lesson.

My wife had followed me from the hall without my noticing. She turned and sprinted into the dining room, returning within seconds with a napkin.

Draping it over the man's mouth and nose, I pinched his nostrils shut and gave two mouth-to-mouth breaths, then resumed CPR compressions. I paused every two minutes for a pulse check, then restarted the cycle of compressions and rescue breathing.

One-person CPR can't be kept up for long. People think they can do it forever. I know I did before this job. But exhaustion comes on quickly, compressions get weaker and decay into ineffective. Rescuers get winded when breathing for two. It is like blowing up balloons with the added stress of trying to save a life. That's why professionals rotate after several cycles of compressions and breaths.

When the unexpected lands on you, you can't waste time questioning, wondering why. What you do to prevail is assess the situation, evaluate risks, decide what must be done, figure out how to do what must be done, and do it.

I searched my brain for ideas—*what can I do by myself with only civilians around? That's it!* Civilians. American Heart Association training videos I endured every year for the past twelve years popped into mind. Those videos had two versions: one for civilians, one for medical staff.

As EMTs, we had to sit through the same two hours of videos year after year. I hated the wasted time. The video for civilians was too simplistic, below our standards of care. For example, civilians are now trained to skip mouth-to-mouth, but EMTs are required to do rescue breathing.

While the civilian videos were too simplistic, the video for professionals was unrealistic. It showed how a doctor and team of six nurses should do CPR in a clean, quiet, stocked hospital room. When on duty, I worked with one partner, not with a team, and our scene could be an interstate lane or a careening ambulance.

Switching into the American Heart Association form, I pointed to one bystander, "You, get an AED (automatic external defibrillator) if you can find one!" Many public buildings now stocked AEDs.

To another, I pointed and said, "You, call 911!"

To a third, "And you, have someone outside to guide the ambulance crew when they arrive!"

Bystanders leaped into action. All they needed were clear instructions and tasks. I even sounded like the narrator in the Heart Association videos as I followed the script verbatim.

Amazingly, a fellow brought an AED in less than a two-minute-CPR-cycle. I opened the unit, grabbed the sticky pads, and stuck them on my patient's chest. Ordering the group to stand back, I called out, "Clear!" The AED analyzed the man's heart rhythm for several seconds. Then the electronic voice announced, "Shock advised."

"Yes!" Shock advised—the best news I could hear. It meant his heart still had electrical activity, and an electric shock might revive the heart.

"CLEAR!" No one was touching the patient, so I pushed the shock button. His body shuddered, and I immediately resumed CPR.

After another two minutes of CPR I paused to let the AED reanalyze the patient. The computerized voice announced, "No Shock Advised."

This was the best or worst message I could hear. It meant either his heart restarted and was beating again, or all electrical activity had stopped when I shocked it. This would be the flat line of death, beyond a reboot.

Checking for a pulse in his neck, his carotid artery pulsed against my finger tips! He's back!

I stopped compressions but continued with mouth-to-mouth because he didn't breathe by himself.

Someone yelled, "The ambulance is here!"

The medics walked in and took over patient care. I reported, "I've done single-person CPR for maybe fifteen minutes. I shocked once with the AED and achieved ROSC. He's still not breathing on his own."

The crew and I rushed the gurney to their unit as I explained, "I'm a paramedic in South Carolina. It never occurred to me I should bring my jump bag on a vacation, or even a face mask."

The local paramedic chuckled, "He's darn lucky you were here. We'll find an opening for you if you ever move to Ohio."

We shook hands, and they drove off Code 3—lights and sirens. As soon as they did, a wave of exhaustion washed over me, leaving me barely able to walk a straight line. This time I had no partner, no one but Ellie and a couple of high school graduates at their fiftieth reunion.

My hands trembled, my legs felt like rubber, but I managed my way back to our table. I told myself *it's just adrenalin; it'll wear off.* Another guest at our table said, "Here, let me buy you a beer."

I wasn't driving, and I'm uncertain if I had more than one. I am certain I didn't pay for any I did have. Several couples joined us, pulling chairs over from nearby tables.

Ellie said, "That's the first time I saw real CPR. I didn't know how violent it is. And you know, I went to school with him."

I replied, "Yes, when you do CPR correctly, you'll hear what sounds like ribs breaking. It usually isn't, but even if it is, living with broken ribs is better than dying with unbroken bones."

Those boring AHA videos had waited in my subconscious until the moment they were needed. That was a big surprise. Another surprise was being the only healthcare professional in a gathering of 150 adults.

Ellie's eyes sparkled, reflecting multi-colored lights from the rotating disco ball above. She couldn't help smiling. Taking her hand, I said, "I didn't know you had followed me. Thank you for the napkin. I glimpsed you flying through those doors, and you still have your gymnast form. Care to dance?"

She smiled, stood, and hand-in-hand we walked to the dance floor. We swayed more than danced. Neither of us could manage much more. She wore White Shoulders, my favorite perfume. It would be our last dance together.

The reunion ended about eleven o'clock. Ellie's friends Bubba and husband Willie drove us back to their house, where sleep evaded, and conversations continued into the wee hours.

I had saved another life. But I hadn't cheated Death. There was no longer an enemy named Death who I had to defeat. There was only death as a natural part of life. Being a paramedic taught me hard lessons. For one, like a captain of a ship does not rule the waves, I do not rule life or death. The captain and I merely try to navigate around hazards when possible, and we suffer the consequences when we cannot.

On our return home to South Carolina, Ellie regaled her sister and friends with reunion stories. She was animated, smiling, her vibrant self. I smiled and laughed with her, not at the stories, but at her joy.

She said, "Seeing so many of my friends, and especially Bubba, was special. And being there while saving a classmate's life was the cherry on top."

It was our last trip together. Ellie fought her cancer for the remaining months of her life. I wondered whether she ever felt bitter that I could save him and not her. I don't believe she did. She wouldn't. A stopped heart differs from cancer which sucks the life out of the body. We can reboot one, not the other. That's the way it works.

In her final weeks, we sat in white rocking chairs on our wraparound front porch enjoying Fall sunsets. I took family medical leave to help her with home treatments and care for Aubri.

One evening she asked, "Are you going to miss EMS after?" We had talked about how I had to stay home after she died to care for Aubri.

"Hey, I'm turning seventy-three and getting too old for EMS, so don't worry about it."

I never lied to Ellie, so I couldn't say I wouldn't miss it. I imagined she felt some guilt about leaving me alone with added burdens. So I tried to lessen that guilt by saying it was fine with me to stop working.

The whole truth was that I was good at my job and would miss it. Sometimes, my hands moved with a skill that was beyond me. I could start an IV bouncing down the road at seventy miles an hour. Once in a while I took part in a miracle, like breathing life back into a stupid kid who tried to hang himself in a bedroom closet.

But there were days, even weeks, when the only calls we got were for drunks who went to sleep on a sidewalk, or for someone who decided after two days of itching and scratching they were a 911 emergency.

Those calls I wouldn't miss, but I would miss the camaraderie of partners who risked their lives every time we worked a crash on the interstate, or went into a dark house, or into a doctor's office where a patient was threatening with a gun.

Ellie spent her final ten days too weak to leave our bed. We lay there, side by side, and remembered stories of shared adventures. Adventures like her last high school reunion. She started slipping away faster and faster. She became as frail as the hummingbirds she loved to feed. On a Wednesday I gave up and called the hospice center to set her up for home care. They came immediately to get us started, to bring oxygen and morphine.

Hours before slipping into a coma two days later, Ellie said to me, "You know, you weren't the cause of your sister Jeannie's death. It just happened. You did everything a nine-year-old could or should do. You made her death have meaning by saving all the lives you did throughout your life. You can't change the past. You can't atone. And you don't need to anyway. I want you to go to your mind's safe place, smile, and thank her. And finally, I want you to take off the responsibility for life and death you've carried on your shoulders all these years. Lay it down and leave it in that safe place."

My only reply: a nod, a hug. I couldn't get any words past the lump in my throat.

Ellie died two days later. After more than twenty-five years together, her hand lay in mine, and she simply exhaled silently one last time.

Emergency medicine taught me to celebrate life rather than rue death. EMS showed me a life is but the flash of a firefly in the evening, the streak of a shooting star in the night. Today, I hear sirens and air horns, and suddenly—in my mind—I am back on the trucks, putting on disposable gloves, watching the GPS on the screen. I am back in it. I am back on the street. I can almost hear the radio traffic.

I had learned the truth about death, learned to acquiesce in Ellie's death without blame or objection. I came to accept her death, but it took four years. It was a dark, ominous, painful time, wanting to die, giving up, drinking into oblivion. But, the blessing of alcoholism was joining AA and seeing the value of my life illuminated. AA, and Aubri, raised me from the tomb of despair. It took those four years before I could fulfill Ellie's instruction to meet Jeannie in my mind and thank her.

Ellie's parting words to me were in a card she left with our daughter to give me after the funeral:

"Thanks for the Adventure—now go have a new one!
Love, Ellie."

Epilogue

As a street medic I learned the ambulance stops three times. The first stop is arrival at the scene of the emergency. The second stop is at the entrance to the emergency room. The third and final stop is when you step out of your last station, after your last call as a street medic. The stop where you hang up your stethoscope for the last time.

When first certified as an EMT I had to use a rear-view mirror to see middle age, an old man in a young person's profession. There was nothing at all special about me.

Thirteen years. I feel radically different from the person I was thirteen years before, when I was first certified as an EMT, still thinking I was going to beat Death. I am the same person, but not thinking the same way. I gained a thick bark of experience during those years; I am older but the same person. I just can no longer think the way I did back then. I was burnished during those years, sanded down to a warrior's state of mind, thinking live or die. I no longer take my eyes off the road for more than a second. I startle at the wail of a siren. I can't laugh at prat falls. I get anxious in a movie scene with someone drinking or texting while driving, or even looking sideways at a passenger to talk. In a public room I sit with my back to a wall, watching each person coming through a door. Is the scene safe, is that person a threat?

Outside my home, I only glance at my phone, I never wear noise cancelling earbuds, I'm always watching for the stampede of zebras. I use peripheral vision at intersections, looking for the driver who isn't paying attention, who is texting, eating, drinking, applying makeup, looking down at the footwells. And always calculating which way to swerve the steering wheel should I need to.

Our species survived for three hundred thousand years, and our ancestors for millions before that, because we always thought the crouching lion could be just behind that bush over there, watching us, waiting.

• • • •

Don't miss out!

Visit the website below and you can sign up to receive emails whenever David Sofi publishes a new book. There's no charge and no obligation.

https://books2read.com/r/B-A-BCWT-OOWYB

BOOKS 2 READ

Connecting independent readers to independent writers.

www.ingramcontent.com/pod-product-compliance
Lightning Source LLC
Chambersburg PA
CBHW021203020426
42331CB00003B/185